"Lani Muelrath's wonderful book is filled with heart and joy. Presenting 'food, fitness, and frame of mind' as the three pillars of health, she shows you how to be full without being fat, while having an environmentally kind and compassionate kitchen. This is one exercise book that understands that you don't have to exercise like a maniac once you get the food right. Highly recommended."

—John Robbins, author, *The Food Revolution*, *Diet for a New America*, and many other best-sellers

"Lani Muelrath's *Fit Quickies* has the diet right. With simple, effective exercises, the powerful message to be less sedentary, and steps for positive change, Lani takes you forward on the path to a better body—and a healthier life."

—John McDougall, MD, author; founder, the McDougall Program

"*Fit Quickies* is everything you ever wanted in a fitness and health program all in one place! You'll find practical exercise suggestions as well as great, easy tips for changing your diet. Lani Muelrath shows you how to power up your menu in exactly the right way. In our studies at the Physicians Committee for Responsible Medicine, we find that these lifestyle changes help our participants lose weight, reverse diabetes, boost heart health, and really change their lives. With Lani's book, you, too, can easily get on the path to great health."

—Neal Barnard, MD, president, Physicians Committee for Responsible Medicine

"With honesty, expertise, and inspiration, Lani Muelrath offers the perfect prescription for a healthier, happier you. *Fit Quickies* is comprehensive, easy, and sure to change your life."

—Rory Freedman, coauthor, #1 *New York Times* best-seller *Skinny Bitch*

"Lani Muelrath's talent and expertise have come together in the freshest health and fitness book available today. She covers brilliantly the pillars of lifestyle medicine that mean so much to more than 50,000 graduates of our Complete Health Improvement Program (CHIP): targeted fitness, sensible eating, and a winning attitude. Empowered and consistently practiced, these same lifestyle principles have helped our graduates shed excess weight, disarm diabetes, lower high blood pressure and cholesterol, and facilitate heart disease reversal. Looking for living life at its best—with resilience, vitality, and joy? Then dig in, embrace, and flourish! You are on your way to radiant health with Lani's easy-to-read and rock-solid book!"

—Hans Diehl, DrHSc, MPH, founder, CHIP and Lifestyle Medicine Institute

"As a dietitian, a runner, and someone who has followed a vegan diet for nearly two decades, I'm thrilled to finally see a one-stop resource that empowers people to meet their highest health potential though diet and exercise. While never losing sight of everyone's capability to achieve a healthy lifestyle, Lani captivates the reader with her own personal and insightful story toward this goal. She brings us along for the ride and prepares us to take the wheel for the long haul."

—Susan Levin, MS, RD, Director of Nutrition Education, Physicians Committee for Responsible Medicine

"Lani Muelrath is a whirlwind of enthusiasm and encouragement, and in *Fit Quickies* she offers you a special invitation to look and feel better, and a sure path to the life you deserve."

—Douglas J. Lisle, PhD, psychologist and coauthor, *The Pleasure Trap*

"I believe that a properly-put-together plant-based, whole-food nutrition plan is the greatest performance advantage an athlete can have. With this book, Lani Muelrath will get you on track. Get ready to reap the many benefits!"

—Brendan Brazier, former pro Ironman triathlete, best-selling author of *Thrive*, and formulator of Vega

"Fitness is a critical component to a healthy lifestyle. In *Fit Quickies*, Lani Muelrath delivers skillful, superb exercise instruction with a fun and effective approach to reshaping your body. She compellingly offers a toolbox to help you succeed at fulfilling your goals for optimal health, fitness, and wellness."

—Julieanna Hever, MS, RD, CPT, host, *What Would Julieanna Do?*; author, *The Complete Idiot's Guide to Plant-Based Nutrition*

"As an exercise physiologist I am adamant about posture and identifying mobility and stability limitations before initiating exercise training. Lani builds a brilliant and attractive model from the ground up, addressing importance of correct body position before and throughout each exercise. Beautifully detailed, comprehensive, an excellent and friendly recipe for your journey to improved health and fitness, *Fit Quickies* inspires you to get serious about changing your body—and gives you the tools to do it."

—Steve Henderson, PhD, Department of Biology and Kinesiology, California State University, Chico; owner, SportFit Performance Training

"Losing weight—and more importantly, true wellness—cannot be achieved and sustained by virtue of fad diets. It requires a comprehensive approach that contemplates the optimum health and harmony of mind, body, and spirit. Lani Muelrath's *Fit Quickies* beautifully embraces this perspective, deftly providing the reader with expert advice to change not just your waistline, but your life—the plant-based way."

—Rich Roll, plant-based ultra-athlete and best-selling author of *Finding Ultra: Rejecting Middle Age, Becoming One of the World's Fittest Men, and Discovering Myself*

FIT
QUICKIES

5-Minute, Targeted
Body-Shaping Workouts

Lani Muelrath

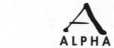

ALPHA

A member of Penguin Group (USA) Inc.

To conscious eating, a fit body, healthy living, and the power you have each and every day to re-create yourself by the way you eat, move, and think. The possibilities!

ALPHA BOOKS

Published by Penguin Group (USA) Inc.

Penguin Group (USA) Inc., 375 Hudson Street, New York, New York 10014, USA • Penguin Group (Canada), 90 Eglinton Avenue East, Suite 700, Toronto, Ontario M4P 2Y3, Canada (a division of Pearson Penguin Canada Inc.) • Penguin Books Ltd., 80 Strand, London WC2R 0RL, England • Penguin Ireland, 25 St. Stephen's Green, Dublin 2, Ireland (a division of Penguin Books Ltd.) • Penguin Group (Australia), 250 Camberwell Road, Camberwell, Victoria 3124, Australia (a division of Pearson Australia Group Pty. Ltd.) • Penguin Books India Pvt. Ltd., 11 Community Centre, Panchsheel Park, New Delhi—110 017, India • Penguin Group (NZ), 67 Apollo Drive, Rosedale, North Shore, Auckland 1311, New Zealand (a division of Pearson New Zealand Ltd.) • Penguin Books (South Africa) (Pty.) Ltd., 24 Sturdee Avenue, Rosebank, Johannesburg 2196, South Africa • Penguin Books Ltd., Registered Offices: 80 Strand, London WC2R 0RL, England

Copyright © 2013 by Lani Muelrath

International Standard Book Number: 978-1-61564-239-7
Library of Congress Catalog Card Number: 2012947182

15 14 13   8 7 6 5 4 3 2 1

Interpretation of the printing code: The rightmost number of the first series of numbers is the year of the book's printing; the rightmost number of the second series of numbers is the number of the book's printing. For example, a printing code of 13-1 shows that the first printing occurred in 2013.

Printed in the United States of America

Note: This publication contains the opinions and ideas of its author. It is intended to provide helpful and informative material on the subject matter covered. It is sold with the understanding that the author and publisher are not engaged in rendering professional services in the book. If the reader requires personal assistance or advice, a competent professional should be consulted.

The author and publisher specifically disclaim any responsibility for any liability, loss, or risk, personal or otherwise, which is incurred as a consequence, directly or indirectly, of the use and application of any of the contents of this book.

Trademarks: All terms mentioned in this book that are known to be or are suspected of being trademarks or service marks have been appropriately capitalized. Alpha Books and Penguin Group (USA) Inc. cannot attest to the accuracy of this information. Use of a term in this book should not be regarded as affecting the validity of any trademark or service mark.

Most Alpha books are available at special quantity discounts for bulk purchases for sales promotions, premiums, fund-raising, or educational use. Special books, or book excerpts, can also be created to fit specific needs. For details, write: Special Markets, Alpha Books, 375 Hudson Street, New York, NY 10014.

CONTENTS

INTRODUCTION

What if I were to hand you several simple, focused, quick exercises specifically designed to target your body's "challenged" spots?

What if I told you you can do these exercises in the privacy of your own home or take them with you on the road anywhere, anytime, with no pricey special equipment or bulky fitness machines necessary?

What if I told you you can say good-bye to obsessive, unhealthy dieting and habits that keep sabotaging your success and finally have the health, shape, energy, and physical confidence you've always dreamed of?

And what if I told you all you had to do to get there was follow a simple, proven plan, without white-knuckle hunger or grueling, disheartening, excessively time-consuming workouts?

And what if I told you I'm inviting you to fall in love with carbs all over again? I'm not going to keep you apart. You were born to be together.

Now do I have your attention?

If you think eating, weight loss, and healthy fitness shouldn't be a constant, confusing struggle, you're right. They shouldn't be, and they aren't, even if it seems you—like me—have spent years trying to prove otherwise. Be confident that radiant health can be yours, no matter what your age or how many times you may have "failed" in the past. You have every reason to feel hope. Perhaps by the time you've read about my journey, you'll see why. And maybe you'll even see a little of yourself in my story.

I know you may feel frustrated. You might even have spent hundreds, if not thousands, of dollars trying to find a "magic bullet" to make your fitness and weight-loss dreams come true. I understand how you feel.

Or maybe you're simply stuck, frustrated with your health and body-shaping plan, floundering around short of your ever-elusive weight-loss goals.

I can help. In the following pages, I help you understand why you haven't succeeded in your previous weight-loss efforts. And more importantly, I show you how to nudge yourself healthfully and happily into that winner's circle. All it may take is a tweak or two to what you're already doing. Along the way, I'm going to share my own diet, exercise, and weight-loss journey.

I've traveled a wearisome, winding road to get to where I am today, where weight management is easy, exercise is fun, and eating is a joy. There's nothing like being fit, trim, energetic, healthy, and well fed. There's nothing like having strength and vitality to make it possible to live large—and I don't mean in size.

My Story

I have a long and colorful diet and exercise history—30 years of constantly battling my weight, being at war with food and with my body, and not having the lasting success or real results I craved, no matter what I did. My weight eventually climbed to a high of almost 200 pounds. Unfortunately, I'm one of those people with a genetic code preset to gain weight easily. The good news, I found, is that with diet and exercise, you can alter the expression of those genes.

But for a long time I couldn't seem to realize the dream I was determined to find: lasting weight loss, resilient energy, great shape, *and* a fully satisfying amount of food on my plate. I couldn't shake the deep conviction that this should be my birthright and that I shouldn't have to be a slave to a diet that kept me hungry or to devote ever-expanding chunks of time to exercise.

And one never came along with the other. If I dieted to lose weight, I didn't have the energy to exercise, and it all fell apart in short order because hunger overcame my dietary resolve. I could exercise, exercise, exercise, running miles every day, yet as I learned—over and over again, despite all my attempts to the contrary—you can't out-train a bad diet.

For decades, I craved a simple solution, but lasting success was always lost in empty diet and exercise promises. Sound familiar?

My Defining Moment

My turning point came more than 17 years ago, when I became exhausted and disheartened from the constant battle. To be honest, I felt like I was at war with my body. I was working full-time during the day, teaching fitness at night, and squeezing in my own workouts while meticulously trying to manage my diet, with intermittent and hard-won results. It had to be my genes or my thyroid—or both—I decided. That must be it!

I even toyed with the idea of resigning myself to being a "fit at any size" person. This wasn't my first choice, but somehow it seemed to be choosing me. Maybe you've even thought the same thing.

Finally, the whole thing reached a tipping point. I walked in the door after a long day at work, zonked from yet another $1\frac{1}{2}$-hour workout at the gym. My gym bag was digging into one shoulder while my case of papers from work carved into the other. I was tired and hungry, and I just wanted to eat, lie down, and sleep.

Here I was, working out hard, but as carefully as I was managing my diet, I was getting diminishing returns. I was essentially eating less, exercising more, and slowly gaining weight anyway. Talk about not fair! What's more, none of it was giving me what I really wanted, which was the pleasure of a fit body with the freedom to *eat*.

At this point, I decided there must be a way to be slim and energetic, enjoy what I ate, exercise a little, and get on with it. I never stopped believing in this possibility. (Perhaps you haven't either. Good.) I had been chronically playing around with diet and exercise and pretty much ending up where I started. I stopped and asked myself, *What am I missing here?*

My 50-Pound Weight Loss

Finally, I achieved success—and on my own terms. My hunger was satisfied, and I developed an approach to exercise that required just reasonable "workout" time. I eventually lost 50 pounds and have kept that weight off for more than a dozen years—at a time in life when everyone else seems to be packing on the fat and racking up the numbers on the scale. And it keeps getting easier for me.

What made the difference? Why success after so many years? What had changed?

The Three Pillars of Successful Body Transformation

I discovered that healthy weight and fitness success has three essential pillars:

- **Exercise:** How you move (or don't move) your body

- **Diet:** What you eat

- **Mind-set:** Your mastery of your psychology

When you get all three in alignment, you're unstoppable. But to get what you want, you have to go three for three, or your success will be limited, lopsided, and easily abandoned.

In this book, we take a closer look at the important fundamentals of each pillar. I share specific details on exactly what to do for healthy fitness in each arena—exercise, diet, and mind-set.

And that's exactly what changed, for me, after so many years. Was it my diet? Yes. Was it my exercise? With the right food in place? Yes. Was it thinking differently? First and foremost, yes.

Perhaps, like me, you've had it with exercise programs with inflated and exaggerated claims. The simple truth is, you have to move your body, challenge it in a variety of ways, and keep doing it. Not only that, but you need to *not sit too much*. The two are independent yet related. Each is so important that, whether you're looking for health and vitality, wanting to take a few inches off your waistline, or seeking to add a few extra years to your life, you need to address both. In the following chapters, I show you exactly what that means and give you simple strategies to make it easy. I share clear guidelines for activity that deliver the results I demand. I teach you 14 Fit Quickies in this book. These 5-minute workout gems make a brilliant addition to your body-shaping and energizing exercise arsenal. You can still do the workouts you enjoy; Fit Quickies add variety, focus, and fun to your usual routine and keep your body guessing—the hallmarks of a solid body-shaping program.

Fit Quickies are perfect for revolutionizing your workouts. These research-driven, physical therapist– and exercise physiologist–approved targeted exercises promise to change the shape of your muscles and restore your strength in a refreshing and innovative format.

Perhaps you, too, are suspicious of the dietary plans that encourage you to eat nutritionally challenged "food," keeping you locked in weight-loss limbo and in total frustration when it comes to getting healthy. The compelling evidence is in: the optimal and easiest pathway to achieving exceptional health and your ideal weight is a whole-food, plant-based diet. This way of eating respects your body's need to be full and your desire to not be fat. In the following chapters, you learn exactly how I eat to easily stay trim, year after year, maintaining my 50-pound weight loss. I show you how you, too, can use these principles along with a simple, time-tested, doctor- and dietitian-approved food plan that won't leave you hungry. If your diet attempts have been focused on portion control or severely restricting carbs, you're doomed and you know it. Help is on the way!

To see a photo history of my weight loss, go to lanimuelrath.com.

When you get the food right, the actions of losing weight, shaping your body, and getting fit and healthy are all so much easier. You carve your figure with your fork. And did you know that the leading cause of death in the United States is nutritionally controllable diseases like heart disease, obesity, certain cancers, and stroke—all diseases we can eat ourselves toward or away from? Undeniable research data show a whole-food, plant-based, low-fat diet is unprecedented in helping you live a healthy, energetic, longer life. At the same time, you reduce environmental impact and create a more compassionate kitchen. How sweet is that?

Plants provide all the proteins, calcium, iron, and other vitamins and minerals your body needs, without the drawbacks of animal products that can weaken your bones, promote cardiovascular or other diseases, or create chronic inflammation. You easily get the complex carbohydrates you need for sustained energy, plus healthy fats that don't clog your circulation, from plant-based sources. What's more, antioxidants and phytonutrients are yours in abundance. My goal is to keep it simple, stick to the basics, and not distract you with supplements, special foods, or concoctions and isolated nutrients.

Finally—and of ultimate importance—when I lost the weight, in addition to the exercise I practiced and the food I put on my plate, I discovered I had to pay attention to what I was thinking and feeling. When making changes, you need to have compassion for yourself and fully support your own endeavors. Without these inner shifts in thinking, the other two pillars of transformation—exercise and diet—are temporary and, at best, superficial. You have to keep in mind what you're looking for. Yes, a slim, energetic, healthy body is one goal, but physical confidence, productivity, fulfillment, and happiness should be, too.

Your fitness, health, and energy are a part of the bigger picture of your life. Your body is the means through which you experience your existence, fulfilling your passion or purpose, contribution, livelihood, avocations, and just plain joy of living. Don't discount the value of this. Don't excuse it away. It's huge and vital to your success.

Acknowledgments

For her vision and belief from the start, thank you to Lori Cates Hand. Thanks to the talented Marilyn Allen and to Bre Whalen. Appreciation to Len Kravitz, PhD, for always taking the time to address my exercise physiology questions. Special thanks to Steve Henderson, PhD, for his hearty support and review of the exercise materials. Thank you to Kelly Guinane, DPT, for meticulously going over each Fit Quickie, and to Clarence Bass, for his spirited enthusiasm and gift of time. I am grateful every day for the foundation in movement with which "Miss H.," my high school dance teacher, infused me. Thank you to my team at Mike Agliolo Productions: Michael Agliolo, Rick Carpenter, Amy Shockley, and Shannon Fuller.

Deep appreciation to John McDougall, MD, for his pivotal role in my personal success in health and life work. His words of advice and encouragement, beginning with "Write about what you know," never failed to inspire. Thank you to Jean Antonello, who absolutely changed my life when it comes to food, eating, and my body.

Appreciation to Matt Lederman, MD, for his expertise and insights about all things food and eating. Thank you to heart-centered hero-of-change psychotherapist Doug Lisle, PhD. Special thanks to the effervescent Julieanna Hever, RD, for her spirited support. Thanks to the very kind and generous John Robbins, Colleen Patrick-Goudreau, and Gene Baur, each of whose work has made an indelible imprint on my life and the direction of my work. Special appreciation for the support and friendship of the team at Physician's Committee for Responsible Medicine: Neal Barnard, MD, Jill Eckart, and the energetic Susan Levin, MS, RD, for her valued assistance in editing the nutrition materials. To Rory Freedman, Hans Diehl, Rich Roll, and Brendan Brazier—your immediate enthusiasm and support means more than you know, thank you. Special thanks to the team in Kinesiology at Butte College: Craig Rigsbee, Mario Vela, Carol Stanley-Hall, Fran Babich, and Kathy Todd, among others.

Thank you to my parents, Chet and Dottie Younghans, who played a crucial part in this book's production by instilling in me, from a very young age, the love of healthy food and an active lifestyle via hiking, camping, and family adventures in the wild. Thanks to my sisters, Pam Younghans and Kristie Foss, who provide an ever-present foundation of support as only sisters can. All for one and one for all.

And most of all, to my husband and the love of my life, Greg. The process of writing a book is not without its extraordinary opportunities and steep learning curves. You've been there with unrivaled guidance, love, and support every step of the way. Thank you.

Special Thanks to the Technical Reviewers

Fit Quickies was reviewed by two experts who double-checked the accuracy of what you'll learn here. Special thanks are extended to Steve Henderson and Susan Levin.

Dr. Henderson teaches human physiology, nutrition for sport and fitness, exercise testing, and prescription and principles of strength and conditioning at California State University, Chico. He also owns SportFit Sport Performance Training, where he works with patient rehab. He is also a national speaker on human movement assessment and kinetic chain dysfunction.

Susan Levin, MS, RD, is the director of nutrition education at the Physicians Committee for Responsible Medicine, a nonprofit organization that advocates for the prevention of disease through a plant-based diet. She is a licensed registered dietitian in the State of New York and in the District of Columbia. She credits her health, love of running, and boundless energy to her 15+ years of practicing what she preaches.

FIT QUICKIE FUNDAMENTALS

Not long after I added what would eventually become the Fit Quickies to my workout routine, my students began asking me what I was doing differently that was creating noticeable differences in my physique. My legs had a new shape, there was a marked lift in my glutes, my arms displayed a new curve, and something different was going on all through my middle. Their questions inspired me to publish an article called "The Forgotten Body Shaping Secret That Gives You Results in the Places You Want Them: Put This Gem into Your Workouts and Watch Your Body Change."

The response was overwhelming. You'd think I'd invented isolation exercise. I didn't—it's been around as long as people have been doing calisthenics and pumping iron. I just made a point of seeking out the best isolate-and-overload muscle moves I could find, tweaked them with valuable muscle-challenging information I discovered in my research on exercise, molded them with my background in exercise form and alignment, and started putting them into practice.

The Story of Fit Quickies

What is the "forgotten body-shaping secret" that gives you results in the places you want them? Isolate and overload, targeting the muscles responsible for changing the shape of your body. Although these exercises had been a regular part of my routine previously, it had been awhile since my workouts had included a regular dose of such targeted work. Yet after a time, I started to miss them—and without them, I wasn't getting quite the body shaping I wanted. I missed the extra something I gained with the deeper muscle challenges they offered. So I began to incorporate them in my workouts again. These exercises became the first in the Fit Quickie collection.

Somehow, in these days of overall conditioning, "gentle" yoga, and functional fitness, this isolate-and-overload technique has gotten lost in the shuffle. Don't get me wrong—you can build a fine, healthy fitness program on general, functional fitness exercise routines. But if you're looking for a little something extra to help create the kind of shape and physical confidence you can achieve with isolate-and-overload challenges, you're going to love Fit Quickies.

Today we have more information about how to effectively use targeted exercises while sparing your joints. We've developed refined techniques to really drive home the challenge—right into the muscle—quicker than ever. And you don't need heavy weights to do it. As I learned in dance class long ago, in most cases, you can do it with your own body weight by the way you position your body, and you can do it by adding a few simple fitness props to offer extra resistance—and fun!

If you really want to change the shape of your body, you need to build muscles—especially those muscles that usually get left out of the action during your daily activities. Targeting muscles specifically for workload gives those muscles more body-shaping opportunity. You go from general to specific. Once you've found them—the muscles that are big players in giving your body great curves and putting extra bounce in your stride—you have to show them you mean business by challenging their current profile. You need to give those muscles the type of work that makes them sit up, take notice, and change shape. The kind of demand that gives your thighs beautiful lines, seriously lifts your seat, and makes your arms solid.

How did this collection of targeted exercises become known as Fit Quickies? It's an important part of the story because it underscores how flexible these exercises really are.

On the way to an adventure at a favorite tropical spot, I wondered how my workout schedule would go while there. Sure, I always get plenty of exercise when we travel, whether walking or hiking or schlepping scuba tanks about, and I get some good cardio kick time swimming to and from the reef. Yet as often as I have great intentions of keeping up with workouts for balancing muscle strength and shape, during travel—especially to tropical locales— it can be too hot to work out. My best-laid plans usually sputter and fade after a few days in the pressing heat.

This time, I decided to try something different. Over the previous months, I had cultivated a growing mental list of some of my body-sculpting and strengthening favorites, drawing upon years of dance training and isolation exercises I'd taught in my conditioning classes. I had discovered that little challenges allowed me to work deep into specific muscles for a fantastic shaping result, but without the lengthy commitment of a full-blown workout. With an assortment of these exercises, I could just pick and choose what I wanted to do each day.

On this particular trip, I selected two or three of these moves each day or two. Some I could do on the floor, watching the palms sway a few feet away. Some I could do with the assist of the kitchen counter as my exercise bar while waiting for my morning hot brew to be ready. Some I could even do against the side of the truck while waiting for my dive buddy to finish loading his gear.

The results were brilliant. Not only did I stay in shape and keep my shape (there is a difference), but I felt invigorated and energetically refreshed in 5 minutes. I loved the feel and instant tightening effect of these isolated, targeted muscle-overload exercises.

I soon realized I could easily take these exercises anywhere and toss them into all kinds of situations—quick little bits of fitness. Thus, the name *Fit Quickies* was born. Drawing upon my years of dance training and surefire exercises from years of coaching and teaching fitness, I focused on the areas of the body that are most neglected yet also responsible for shaping the body and giving a graceful stride: abs, triceps, inner thighs, gluteals, hamstrings, and quads. I added my own intensifying elements and consulted with a physical therapist to optimize them for safety. I even began combining them into effective bundles—because I *knew* this was going to be something others would love, too. My 7 *Seconds to a Flat Belly* video became the perfect starting point for Fit Quickies and proudly holds the title of Fit Quickie #1.

Fast-forward to today. The Fit Quickies collection has expanded and now includes a growing list of targeted muscle-shaping and strengthening moves—14 of these are included in this book. Fit Quickies continue to form the foundation of my travel and at-home targeted body-shaping exercises. And now you can use them to shape your body, too.

The Principles of Fit Quickies

At the core of the Fit Quickies are three main ideas:

- Position precisely

- Isolate

- Overload

Proper positioning places the workload on the specific muscles you're targeting, inviting the muscle shaping you're looking for. It also takes the heavy lifting off your joints. If you wonder why your current workout isn't giving you the body shaping you desire, you now might have some insights into why—and the tools with which to work for change.

 Comprehensive movement and exercise routines that promote your body's overall wellness also play an important role. They improve your health, enhance your muscle balance, and cultivate your ability to operate with vitality.

And if changing the shape of your body is on your goals list, you've got to make the principles of isolate and overload important elements of your training. Be sure that, within your exercise routine, you're placing enough demand on those lazy muscles—a demand that will force them to change.

The P.A.I.R. Principles

Before we get started with these powerful moves, we need to address some quick tips and pointers on setup for all Fit Quickies that make a big difference in your results. You'll simply be applying the three core principles mentioned earlier with specific actions. I've taken all the guesswork out of it so you can get best results right from the start.

All Fit Quickies launch with a specific sequence I call P.A.I.R.:

- Position

- Anchors

- Isolation

- Repetitions

Let's take a close look at each of these.

P: Position

Each Fit Quickie is to be performed with respect to the integrity of correct anatomical alignment. This means your first goal is to get your body correctly positioned before you begin.

Any worthwhile movement system prioritizes good posture. I learned this long ago from my high school dance teacher, who had studied with Martha Graham. Miss H., as we called her, taught me everything there was to know about posture, carriage, the core, and fluidity of movement. I can hear her voice when I exercise: "Upright your spine! Lift your ribs from your hips, shoulders back, chest open, extend the top of your head to the ceiling—and pull those stomach muscles in!" To this day, I thank her for the foundation of my love and study of exercise, movement, physical culture, and its power to transform our bodies, our energy, our minds, our physical confidence, and our lives.

Correct anatomical alignment places your body in the best position for protecting and restoring good posture, as well as safeguarding your joints. It also brings all your muscles into play right away and delivers focus, energy, and, yes, grace to each move. Fit Quickies are more than body shapers. They also bring an elegance and energy to your workouts that carries through to the rest of your day—that's how I designed them. Getting your muscles and bones all lined up for action before you start sets you up for precision of movement. It allows you to make Fit Quickies even quicker and more effective so you can get more accomplished in less time. Fewer well-done repetitions trump a higher number of less-focused moves—every time.

It's vital that you anchor your body for exercise by engaging key postural muscles. Today we call them "core" muscles; back then, we just called them abdominals, backs, and glutes. You'll see this foundation reflected and reinforced in the setup of each Fit Quickie. Eventually, I hope you'll automatically remember to line up your body into optimal posture, including what I call *anchored neutral:* your shoulders stacked over your hips, your chest open, your neck long, your abdominals braced, your back in its natural functional curve—and your gluteals in gear.

Your vertebral column has three natural curves: cervical (neck), thoracic (middle), and lumbar (lower back). *Neutral spine* usually refers to the lumbar area. It's a pain-free position of the lumbar spine attained when the pressures in and around the pelvis joint structures are evenly distributed and the pelvis is balanced between its anterior and posterior positions, according to Len Kravitz, PhD, and Ken Fowler in a 2011 report for *IDEA Health and Fitness*. This is the strongest position for the spine when you're standing or sitting, and the one within which you're meant to move. Adding resistance exercise, however, demands you call in reinforcements to help maintain your natural curves. That's where *anchored neutral* comes in.

Poor alignment often shows up as excessive anterior pelvic tilt. This means that the top of your pelvis is tipped too far forward, lifting your tailbone posteriorly, resulting in an exaggerated curve in your lumbar region. This position releases your abdominals and puts pressure on your lower back, which can lead to back pain and a host of other problems.

In contrast, in proper functional anatomical alignment, as shown in the following photo, the pelvis is aligned correctly beneath the shoulders and all the back's natural curves are intact. This position normally includes only a slight anterior pelvis tilt and is the position you want your body in as you move through your day. Your head is held high on a lifted extension from your spine, your chest is open, your shoulders are back, and your gaze is forward.

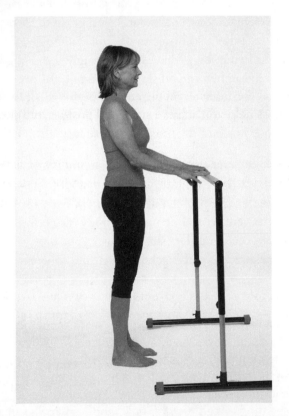

A spine in neutral position respects the natural curves of the spine. Anchor neutral position by engaging your core to create a strong foundation for exercise.

From this position—neutral spine—it's a small, simple, yet important step to create *anchored* neutral, where your abdominal, back, and gluteal muscles are activated to brace your core and provide support for all movement. To achieve the anchor, engage your abdominals, gently lifting the weight of your ribs directly from your hips to upright your spine. Secure your shoulder blades on your back, and tighten through your gluteals to stabilize the position of your pelvis, while keeping the natural, neutral curves through your spine.

This muscle activation offsets any tendency to release your pelvis into excessive anterior tilt as you exercise by strongly rooting its position. Anchored neutral is the position in which you begin all Fit Quickies. (If you've had dance or Pilates training, you'll recognize this position.) I remind you through the course of each exercise to be mindful of protecting and regaining anchored neutral as you move.

A: Anchors

With each Fit Quickie, you'll establish specific anchor points in addition to your abdominals and gluteals. These anchors help you achieve sustained posture and position. They also enable you to more accurately isolate the muscles you're targeting with each exercise.

Your anchor could be the light touch of your hand on a counter or dance bar, your knee on a bench, or your hip and hand on the carpet. With each exercise, I describe your anchor points so you can get in the habit of paying attention to them, right along with position, to make your Fit Quickies a joy to complete correctly and effectively.

I: Isolate

Remember, Fit Quickies intertwine the concepts of isolation and overload. Isolating certain muscles means you can specifically create an overload on them to build strength, balance, and beautiful shape.

One of the reasons the Fit Quickies are so effective at shaping your body is that they force into play the muscles that have a dramatic impact on your shape—muscles that likely have been neglected or underactivated for some time. In our daily lives, we easily establish and repeat patterns of movement that allow the stronger, more dominant muscles to keep prevailing with the workload. No wonder so many people's abs and inner thighs are out of shape—these muscles checked out of the program long ago because they weren't being sufficiently challenged.

With the isolate factor of Fit Quickies, you put thought to body using focus and precision, and command those important structural muscles back into play.

R: Repetitions

When you're correctly lined up and in position, and have your anchors in place, you're ready to begin the sequence of repetitions that make up each Fit Quickie. Each exercise has its own unique sequence of repetitions, although you'll see some patterns emerge. You'll also see instructions for modifying exercises, how to increase the challenge as you progress, and suggestions for how to increase the challenge.

 Listening to music has been proven to make workouts easier and more effective. In fact, it's been shown to increase endurance by as much as 15 percent, as reported by A. Szabo and colleagues in the *Journal of Sports Medicine and Physical Fitness* in 1999. Music can distract you from fatigue, ramp up your motivation, improve your coordination, and increase your sense of relaxation. As the beat drives harder, you push harder—without even thinking about it. You can use your favorite tunes or download a soundtrack I composed for use with Fit Quickies at fitquickies.com. Let the beat connect with and inspire your inner dancer, and watch your strength and endurance soar.

I know you're excited to get started. But before introducing you to the Fit Quickies, I want to be sure you have everything you need to know to create a solid fitness program of which the Fit Quickies form an important part. Of course, feel free to peek ahead and start sneaking in your favorite Fit Quickies today.

THE EXERCISE PRESCRIPTION

There's no getting around it: regular physical exercise—beyond simply going about your daily living activities—is essential to improving and maintaining healthy vitality as well as shaping a body you're happy to be in. But how much exercise do you really need? What's the best kind of exercise to do? Where do you start? And how can you fit it into your busy schedule? Let's begin with what exercise will do for you and take it from there.

Why Exercise?

Our bodies are designed to move, walk, run, jump, and play. The problem is, we're biologically programmed, since our earliest ancestors, to conserve our energy for the saber-tooth-tiger emergency that never comes. We've created so many shortcuts to make life easier, we don't get nearly enough of the exercise we need for resilient, dynamic health. And we've invented so many step-savers, we're seriously short on taking steps altogether. This saves us all kinds of trouble, but at the same time creates all kinds of other trouble for our health and beltlines. Our biology has simply not kept up with our technology.

People think that just because I'm "in fitness," I always love to work out. Not true. Often I move past the urge to take it easy by keeping in mind what I know is a far greater reward: a well-exercised body. What gets me going, one workout after another, is the way I feel when I'm done; the way I feel each morning as I spring out of bed with supple, conditioned muscles; the way I feel when I'm a few heartbeats into a workout; and the mental resurrection that comes as a result of the exertions of getting back into my body. The satisfaction of meeting a physical challenge gets me going, time and time again.

Think about it. Don't you always feel more energized, focused, confident, vital, and motivated to make healthy choices after you exercise? Of course you do. Use that feeling to get yourself going on that first rep, that first lift, that first step or push on the pedal.

The number-one reason to exercise is not because it burns calories, but because of what it does for your brain, biochemistry, and physical confidence. That's not to mention developing a strong, shapely body; reversing disease biomarkers; gaining radiant energy; and crafting a body that just plain works better.

The Benefits of Exercise

Exercise has a tremendous positive impact on your health and well-being. It …

- Improves your body composition by reducing fat weight and increasing muscle mass.

- Enhances enzymatic action that discourages fat storage.

- Improves your blood lipid profile—triglycerides and cholesterol—and reduces your risk of coronary heart disease.

- Reduces your risk of type 2 diabetes and improves insulin sensitivity and glucose metabolism.

- Lessens your risk of stroke, combats osteoporosis, and reduces the incidence of some cancers.

- Keeps your musculoskeletal system primed.

- Combats arthritis by improving aerobic capacity, muscle strength, and joint and functional ability.

- Reduces stress and anxiety and improves your mood, confidence, self-esteem, and overall mental outlook.

- Helps you cut down on smoking and also alcohol and caffeine consumption.

- Increases your desire to eat healthier, helps get your emotions under control, and aids in personal productivity.

Exercise turns out to be the closest thing to a wonder drug … scientists have discovered. … It not only relieves ordinary, everyday stress, but it's as powerful an antidepressant as Prozac.

—Kelly McGonigal, *The Willpower Instinct*

Quick Self-Assessment

When putting the many benefits of exercise into place in your life, it helps to take an honest appraisal of how the state of your health is right now. Ask yourself some questions to assess where you are and where you want to go, starting with these:

- What aspect of my current state of health makes me unhappy but could be positively affected by regular exercise?

- What exactly do I want to change about my health and my body, and why?

- Am I avoiding certain situations that involve physical activity?

- Am I able to carry a bag of groceries from the car to the kitchen, for example, with ease?

- Am I easily winded, finding myself breathless when I go about everyday tasks?

- Are my clothes tighter than they were last year?

- Am I finding it harder to turn my head to safely back out of a parking space?

The answers to these questions are indicators of your current state of health, fitness, strength, cardiorespiratory endurance, and flexibility. They are concrete connections that provide you with powerful reasons for change and give purpose to your exercise plan. You need the *why* first. Armed with this information, you're better able to set goals for improving your fitness.

Bodybuilder, fitness expert, and author Clarence Bass is one of my all-time favorites in the fitness world, and his early books were among the first on my exercise and fitness bookshelf. I asked Bass to recommend a self-assessment tool for use home to gauge physical fitness. Without skipping a beat, he said, "The first is the mirror. The second is how your clothes fit."

For a more formal assessment, you can make an appointment at a local gym for some baseline fitness measurements, but that's not always a practical or possible option. Luckily, assorted fitness tools and calculators are readily available online to help you conduct a variety of assessments, such as body mass index (BMI), percent body fat, weight training load, physical activity calorie calculator, and risk of chronic disease. Establishing health and fitness baselines gives you specifics you can use to create concrete goals and then measure your progress.

For a list of free helpful fitness assessment tools and calculators, log on to lanimuelrath.com.

Setting Long- and Short-Term Goals

The long-term fitness goals you establish should be straightforward and specific and should emphasize what you want to accomplish. They should be a little bit of a stretch from your current norm, but not entirely out of reach. For example, you could set a goal of dropping one pants size, being able to briskly move for more than a mile without a break, or being able to lift 20 pounds. Also allow yourself sufficient time to obtain your desired results. Setting goals gives meaning and purpose to your exercise and diet plan.

If, for example, your clothes are tighter than they were last year and you're not happy about that, one of your long-term goals could be to improve your body composition—your fat-to-lean ratio. You can monitor this specifically with body fat calculations or with a simple measuring tape. Or if you're easily winded and want to change that, one of your long-term goals could be to become more aerobically fit.

From your list of long-term goals, you create short-term goals, or objectives. These are the definitive actions you take each day to move closer toward your long-term goals. This is where it all happens! For example, to meet a long-term goal of improving your body composition, you could set short-term goals of addressing specific aspects of your daily nutrition and also becoming less sedentary to decrease your body fat stores. To reach a long-term goal of becoming more aerobically fit, you could do more cardiorespiratory exercise each week to build your aerobic fitness. The more specific you are in establishing your short-term daily action goals, the better.

Examples of specific short-term daily action goals are to walk for 15 minutes every day or practice a strength-training routine two or three times this week. Short-term goals can be accomplished realistically within a brief period of time. For example, if you've been totally inactive for some time, you might start by setting a short-term goal to walk during lunch for 10 minutes each day for the next week. This short-term goal is an example of a SMART goal.

SMART goals are …

> **Specific:** The planned activity has been clearly defined—walk 10 minutes at lunch.

Measurable: At week's end, you can reflect on whether you walked each day as planned.

Action based: The goal focuses on exactly what you'll be doing.

Realistic: Is it convenient? You need to be able to look at the short-term goal and honestly say, "I can do that!"

Time anchored: The goal is connected with a specific time frame—this week.

Compared to the more ambiguous "I want to get in better shape," SMART goals are specific and measureable. If you can measure it, you can manage it. Setting such goals gives you the feedback you need to see whether you're on track. You can check them off on a chart as "Done!"

How Much Exercise Do You Need?

With all the workouts, specialized exercise equipment, and hype out there, where do you turn to find out exactly what kind and how much—or how little—exercise you need to do each week to be healthy?

Recently, C. Garber and team at the American College of Sports Medicine (ACSM)—the gold standard of fitness research—released the updated ACSM Position Stand. This 2011 document is a comprehensive guideline on exercise, with data culled from more than 400 publications such as scientific reviews, epidemiological and clinical studies, meta-analyses, consensus statements, and more to "present evidence-based direction to developing exercise programs for healthy adults." The report offers recommendations in four areas of exercise: resistance training, cardiorespiratory training, flexibility training, and neuromotor training (the new kid on the fitness block).

Don't worry, I'm not going to ask you read the entire report. Instead, I've pulled together the main points outlining what a healthy exercise schedule might look like. You can compare the information in the following sections to your current physical activity to see whether what you're doing is adequate, get some tips on what to tweak to reach your goals, and learn some key points to keep in mind if you're just getting started.

Always check with your health-care provider to be sure you're healthy enough to start an exercise program and find out about any precautions you need to take as you change your level of activity.

Cardiorespiratory Training

According to the 2011 ACSM Position Stand, cardiorespiratory exercise—or *cardio*, as it's more commonly called—is "purposeful, continuous, rhythmic exercise involving the major muscle groups." Think walking, biking, swimming, running, skiing, jumping, elliptical, aerobics—exercises that challenge your cardiorespiratory system. No stop-and-start exercises.

There's a little flexibility when it comes to the aerobic exercise guidelines, but they're all based on the variables of duration and intensity of exercise. The harder you work, the less time you need to invest. Conversely, the lower the intensity, the more time you should devote. For example, you could do moderate-intensity aerobic exercise for 30 to 60 minutes at least 5 times a week, opt for some higher-intensity work for 20 minutes 3 times per week, or put together a combination of these.

A word about intensity: what's *moderate* intensity, and what does *vigorous* intensity mean? Several methods of measurement can be utilized to assess, but right now, you need a simple one you can count on to ensure you're getting the right intensity for your goals.

Two easy-to-use at-home tools are available for measuring cardiorespiratory intensity, the Borg Rate of Perceived Exertion (RPE) Scale and the even simpler "talk test." You can use both to come up with a pretty good idea of the intensity at which you need to exercise.

With the Borg RPE Scale, it might look like the measure of intensity is quite objective. It is. You're using your body as the feedback tool for measuring "moderate" versus "vigorous" exertion. The following table illustrates the Borg Scale.

Borg Rate of Perceived Exertion Scale

INTENSITY RATING	DESCRIPTION
6	No exertion, such as sitting and relaxing
7	Extremely light, such as standing
8	
9	Very light, such as casual walking
10	
11	Light; comparable to the intensity you experience in a light warm-up
12	
13	Somewhat hard; workout intensity feels mildly challenging
14	
15	Hard (heavy); workout intensity feels difficult
16	
17	Very hard; exercise is at a very demanding intensity
18	
19	Extremely hard; this rigorous intensity cannot be sustained for long
20	Maximal exertion: running from fire

Adapted from: Borg, G. (1973). Perceived exertion: a note on "history" and methods. Medicine and Science in Sports and Exercise. *Volume 5 (Number 2), 90–93.*

The "talk test," in comparison, is just what it sounds like: you observe how well you're able to talk, out loud, while engaging in an activity. The higher the intensity of your workout, the sooner you'll have to stop talking to take a breath, according to R. Persinger and colleagues in a 2004 article in *Medicine and Science Sports and Exercise.*

For example, during a brisk walk, if you can easily recite "Mary Had a Little Lamb" from "Mary" to "… the lamb was sure to go," you're working slightly above couch-potato intensity, or somewhere between 6 and 8 on the Borg Scale.

If you can get as far as "… its fleece was white as snow" before you need to take a breath, your Borg Scale intensity jumped to a 9 or 10 on the scale, or light.

However, if you have to take a breath between phrases like this: "Mary had a little lamb [breath] its fleece was white as snow [breath]," you're probably working at Borg Scale 12 or 13, moderate to somewhat hard.

If you need to take a breath after every word—"Mary" [breath] "had" [breath]—you're working at a vigorous intensity, or Borg Scale 14 to 17.

If talking is a breeze, you want to pick up the pace. If you're gasping for breath to speak, scale back the intensity.

To meet the cardiorespiratory guidelines, aim for moderate-intensity aerobic exercise (Borg Scale 12 or 13) for 30 to 60 minutes at least 5 times a week, or higher-intensity exercise (Borg Scale 14 to 17) for 20 minutes 3 times per week, or a combination of the two. As you become more fit, you can increase the pace of your activity to keep yourself challenged.

 You can compress your cardio time by implementing interval training. I've put together a free how-to guide on interval training, available at lanimuelrath.com.

By assessing your current abilities with these measures of intensity, you'll be able to set your SMART goals for cardiorespiratory training, working your way up to the suggested guidelines for time in training each week.

Resistance Training for Strength

Many people are turned off by the idea of resistance training because they believe they're going to have to lift heavy weights and use all kinds of special equipment to reach their strength and body-shaping goals. Not so. In this book, I've cut through the chaos to make simple, usable sense out of weights and repetitions guidelines so you can get going, quickly and easily, with building a strong, beautiful body.

Here are the ACSM recommended guidelines for resistance training:

- Target the major muscle groups two or three times a week.

- Rest your muscle groups for 48 hours before challenging them again.

- Work at an intensity of 40 percent (beginner) to 70 percent (intermediate) of your 1-repetition max (1-RM) for strength.

- Shoot for 8 to 20+ repetitions.

Your 1-repetition max (1-RM) is the heaviest weight you can lift for 1 repetition.

You might be scratching your head after reading that list. Often a lot of confusion surrounds resistance training, and these guidelines don't do much to quell that. The ranges for intensity and repetitions seem very broad, for example, and percentage of maximum formulas often end up scaring off some people. Testing for maximums isn't an easy or necessarily safe thing to do.

Confusion is compounded by one of the most often-debated topics in the gym: which is better to make muscle, light weight and high reps, or heavy weight and low reps? If you want to "shape" muscle, should your workouts ideally utilize light resistance and high repetitions? And if you want to go for more strength and size, should you cut down on the reps and amp up the weights?

Bulking up doesn't just happen by accident; it's in your genes. Genetic factors are the biggest players in muscular responses to resistance training. Both men and women have to work hard to gain muscle—and women even more so than men, due to hormonal differences. Smaller in size and with lower levels of testosterone, women simply don't have the genetic potential to bulk up the way men do. What women may perceive as bulk is generally fat layered into as well as blanketed over the muscle subcutaneously, or situated under your skin. Both of these types of fat deposit obscure muscle shape. Your hard-won muscles aren't going to show unless you're lean enough.

Heavier weights may still be the best choice for power-lifters when training for explosive power at higher resistance. (Olympic competitors, take note!) Other than that, it turns out, resistance training both with lighter weights and higher repetitions and with heavier weights and lower repetitions produces similar muscular strength responses, as cited in 2008 by Ralph Karpinelli of Adelphi University in New York. Either approach maximizes your genetic potential. "Our data provides further support that low-load contractions performed with numerous repetitions or high-load contractions performed for fewer repetitions will result in similar training induced gains in muscle hypertrophy as previously suggested, or even superior gains" report Nicholas Burd and his team from McMaster University, Ontario, in 2010.

According to the 2010 research findings of the American Council on Exercise, the best way to stimulate and build the maximum number of muscle fibers is to ensure that you meet the following two guidelines:

Use a resistance that gives you maximum effort by the end of the set. You can achieve this either by positioning, using weights, or combining these factors. Maximum effort means you've about reached your limit in terms of doing another repetition, in proper form, with your muscles being challenged. Your set comes to a close not because you're winded or don't want to continue, but because the muscles you're focusing on have reached maximum effort, as corroborated by Karpinelli and Burd.

Your exercise routine fatigues your muscle within the limits of the anaerobic energy system. Specifically, that means within about 90 seconds of effort. For strength, your time frame and intensity should be under 2 minutes.

So you can go either way:

- **Low weights, high reps:** Be sure you max out with the targeted muscle(s) in about 90 seconds or less.

- **High weights, low reps:** You'll achieve muscle overload sooner than in the 90 seconds.

Forget heavy, think effort. It's not the weight; it's the effort you put in by the end of the set.

—Clarence Bass

If higher weights do the trick in less time, should you opt for that? There may be good reason to select the higher rep/low weight option:

Orthopedic concerns. Heavier weights can pose more risk and challenge to your joints.

Access to equipment. At-home fitness workout routines don't always grant the luxury of a full arsenal of heavier weights.

Workout style preferences. Some people prefer the muscle feel of higher repetition work. It becomes quite clear when your muscles are reaching their capacity for challenge, and you learn to seek it. I find higher reps (12 to 15 and up) quite relaxing, very effective, easier on my joints, and safe.

The need for variety. Changing up your workout routine keeps your muscles guessing, and when it comes to shaping your physique, that's a good thing. So mix it up!

What about that suggested 48-hour rest time? And how do you know when you're working too hard—or not hard enough?

According to exercise physiologist Steve Henderson, PhD, you should experience some tightness or soreness along with noticeable fatigue the day after you exercise in the muscles you trained as an indicator your muscles were sufficiently challenged. If you don't feel anything the day after your resistance training workout, chances are, you didn't challenge yourself hard enough and you need to up the intensity next time out.

 When it comes to fitness, higher repetitions to fatigue is the place to land.

—Steve Henderson, PhD

As a rule of thumb, deep challenges to the large muscle groups—hips and legs, chest, and back—often requires a 48-hour rest and recovery period. Smaller muscle and isolation exercises may require a little less time—more like 24 hours. You may still feel some residual tightness and light soreness, but it'll also feel good to work on these muscles within a day. If, on the other hand, you've worked so hard you can't sit or stand properly for a few days, it's time to back off a bit on intensity.

Keep in mind that your recovery time and resiliency will change as you become more overall fit. Beginning exercisers will feel the steepest challenge and have the greatest demand for recovery time. Six weeks into a resistance training program, however, you'll bounce back faster. It's a sign you're becoming stronger and more fit.

Here are some points to keep in mind:

- You build muscle by overloading its current capacity.

- The harder you work the muscle, the more muscle fibers you fire up.

- The amount of resistance used is trumped by the amount of effort experienced within the set.

- To achieve changes in muscle strength, you should complete each set within 90 seconds. A set doesn't have to take the full 90 seconds, but it shouldn't take longer.

- Challenge your muscles by mixing up the amount of resistance and the angle against gravity at which you work the muscle.

- For optimal results, infuse your workouts with variety so you don't do the same sequences week after week. Your body and brain quickly adapt to these patterns, and both respond to novelty with positive progress in strength, ability, and agility.

 Creating a single prescription of an "optimal" resistance training programs isn't and will never be an exact science. Too much variation exists in how different individuals respond to training. However, resistance training at lower resistance and higher repetitions is just as effective in stimulating muscle growth as training with higher resistance and fewer repetitions, confirm Nicholas Burd and associates at McMaster University.

The bottom line? Find the resistance training that you enjoy and that challenges your muscles deeply yet safely by the end of your set. And keep training!

Flexibility Training

Stretching and staying flexible are important components of fitness and well-being. And believe it or not, they're also critical for top-notch body-shaping.

Plus, staying flexible helps protect you from injury. After all, what's going to save you in a fall if not your ability to bend, reach, and otherwise go with the flow?

Here are the ACSM guidelines for flexibility training:

- Target the major muscle groups two or three times a week with stretching.

- Stretch to the point of slight discomfort or feeling of tightness in the muscle.

- Opt for 2 to 4 repetitions of each stretch, for a total of 30 to 60 seconds stretching time per target muscle group. Holding a stretch for 20 to 30 seconds at the point of tightness or slight discomfort enhances joint range of motion, with little apparent benefit resulting from longer durations.

Keep in mind that you may—and should, actually—be doing flexibility training as part of your resistance training. Those hamstring stretches you do after Fit Quickie #4? Flexibility training. The quadriceps stretch after Fit Quickie #6? Flexibility training. The chest stretch after pushups? You get the idea. A stretch or release is provided with each Fit Quickie.

Neuromotor Training

Neuromotor exercise focuses on balance, agility, and coordination—think yoga, tai chi, qigong, and physical therapies. This type of training improves stabilizing muscle strength, gait, and coordination and reduces the risk of falls. For these reasons, it's high on the recommended list of exercise for older adults. Although more data is needed before specific recommendations can be confirmed, there is enough evidence in the research to prompt the ACSM to suggest incorporating 20 minutes on two or more days per week of neuromotor activities, especially for older adults.

Activities you may be practicing in the other three categories may have crossover application in neuromotor training. For example, yoga practices vary widely, and some techniques are oriented to really challenge strength, making them technically a form of resistance training while also a neuromotor exercise. This is where individualizing your workout rotation comes into play. Consider the possibilities!

How to Use the Exercise Guidelines

Do you have to follow the ACSM guidelines to the letter in all four categories? Is it all or nothing? The short answer is "no." Rather, it's an evidence-based guide. You can—and should—modify your exercise plan according to your own physical abilities, health status, exercise responses, and specific goals. And if you're unable or unwilling to meet the exercise targets outlined here, you can still benefit from engaging in exercise, even if it's less than what's recommended. You can always work your way up.

I know you're ready to get going. And if you're already doing regular exercise, seize the inspiration of the moment to balance your workout rotations. But before you do, we have a couple important points to go over: if you're coming off a long period of inactivity or minimal workout time, be cautious about how you start out. Don't jump into a full workout following the ACSM guidelines on Day 1. Instead, start where you are and progress from there. The Fit Quickies are perfect for helping you do just that.

Also think about your current activity and workout schedule. Does it give you everything you need? If not, assess the guidelines to see where you might be able to create a better routine. For example, maybe you're really good at your cardiorespiratory workouts, but it's been a couple years (or more) since you lifted a weight or did a pushup. In that case, you'd want to start building up your resistance-training routine. Or what if you can't remember the last time you stretched your hamstrings? Time to focus on some flexibility.

The only way to become stronger, fitter, better shaped, and more energetic is to step up your physical challenge. You'll greatly enhance your physical and mental health, as well as quality of life, as a result. So create a plan and get started.

Fit Quickies and the ACSM Guidelines

Where do the Fit Quickies fit in with the exercise recommended in the guidelines (resistance training, cardiorespiratory training, flexibility training, and neuromotor training)?

Most of all, Fit Quickies are resistance training with a flexibility component because each Fit Quickie comes with a follow-up stretch. Some Fit Quickies also sneak into the neuromotor category by challenging balance and coordination.

More than anything, it's important to vary your resistance training. You keep your body strong and shapely by asking it to step up to varied challenges. You can combine several Fit Quickies as a resistance workout on their own, or pepper them into your other workouts. Mix it up and have fun with it. Elsewhere in the book, I give you a few suggestions for some of my favorite Fit Quickie combinations I've found particularly effective in making beautiful muscle and a stronger body. And I show you how easy it is to create fun and effective combinations of your own.

Remember, your genetics determine the shape and size potential of your muscles. Yet like just nearly everything else about your body, your actions determine the expression of those genes. You likely have more potential for muscle shape than you're enjoying right now, based on how you challenge your muscles. When you isolate key muscles, bring them into play by recruiting them for action, and provide them with a sustained—although short and intense—workload, your muscles scramble to adapt. The challenge moves deep into your muscle, exhausting your muscle fibers' ability to sustain the targeted exercise and inspiring change.

Only when the demand placed upon it exceeds the muscle's current ability does it rush to build new protein strands—called myofibrils—and increase their thickness and number. New myofibrils allow your muscle to accept the challenge of on the new workload. This is building muscle, and muscle is what shapes and strengthens your body. Plus—and this is a biggie—finding muscle-challenging moves you enjoy doing makes it far more likely that you'll actually do them.

Too Much Sitting Is Hazardous to Your Health

When it comes to physical activity, there are two parts to the health and fitness picture. One is the specific exercises and workouts you do to stay healthy and in shape. The other may surprise you: it's simply to *not* sit too much.

It's true: too much sitting is hazardous to your health. And no, sitting too much is not the same as exercising too little. The good news is, it's an easy fix.

The Problem

As far back as the seventeenth century, physicians noted the relationship between sedentary behavior and poor health. We now know without a doubt that inactivity has its own set of special effects on metabolism, physical function, and health outcomes. Apparently, it's not enough to work out. You also need to take a serious look at how long you spend sitting and reclining.

Not long ago, when we referred to someone as *sedentary*, it meant that person didn't get much physical activity. So if, for example, you were exercising for an hour or so a day, you could call yourself physically active. But this view is changing rapidly as researchers discover that sedentary time is positively correlated to health risk—*regardless of how much physical activity you get in every day*. In this case, *positive* isn't good.

Sedentarism refers to prolonged engagement in sedentary behaviors such as sitting and other activities that require little to no physical movement. A *sedentarist* is someone who spends extended periods of time without moving. An *active couch potato* is someone who does their workouts and then sits all for extended periods the rest of the time.

The Damaging Effects of Sedentary Behavior

Recent evidence suggests that sedentary behavior has a direct influence on metabolism, bone mineral content, and vascular health. It also leads to the following—all of which increase the risk for type 2 diabetes and coronary heart disease—independent of any exercise you do:

- Increased triglyceride levels

- Decreased levels of high-density lipoprotein (HDL) cholesterol—the "good" cholesterol

- Decreased insulin sensitivity

- Metabolic syndrome

- Suppressed lipoprotein lipase (LPL)

LPL is tasked with extracting particles of fat in your blood and transporting them to one of two places: your fat cells for storage, or your muscle cells for energy. Physical activity slows the LPL in fat tissues, making it harder for you to store fat, and increases LPL activity in the skeletal muscle, pushing fat into the muscle cells to be used for energy. The latter is where you want your fat to go.

Physical *inactivity*, on the other hand, does the opposite: it increases your body's LPL activity in the fat tissue and slows it in the muscles. The result? You store fat more easily. *Not* what you're shooting for here.

To examine the effect of complete bed rest on metabolic health, in 2007 Naomi Hamburg and her colleagues at Boston University Medical Center conducted a study of 22 adult volunteers. The participants stayed in bed for more than 23.5 hours a day, getting only 30 minutes a day for bathroom breaks. At the end of the study, although the subjects had no changes in body weight, they experienced significant jumps in total cholesterol, triglycerides, glucose, and insulin resistance. How many days do you think it took for these bed-resters to achieve these results? *Five days!*

What's more, changes in carbohydrate metabolism were sharp. Participants experienced a 67 percent greater insulin response to a glucose load after the 5 days. This suggests that an extended period of sedentary behavior can lead to a dramatically increased metabolic risk. This sedentary physiology needs to be considered distinctly separate from exercise physiology, according to a 2010 report by Mark Tremblay and associates at the Eastern Ontario Research Institute.

 Carbohydrate metabolism is the breakdown of carbohydrates into smaller units your body can use for energy.

Other studies have delivered similar results. In 1998, Ryoki Yanagibori and his team at the University of Tokyo found that 20 days of bed rest resulted in a significant rise in plasma triglycerides and a big drop in HDL cholesterol (the "good" cholesterol). These findings are further corroborated by reports suggesting that people with spinal cord injuries—who spend large amounts of time sedentary—also suffer from an increased risk of cardiovascular disease, as observed by William Bauman and his research team at Veterans Affairs Medical Center in New York in 2008.

Does it matter how many stretches of sedentary time you have in the day? No doubt. We don't know the exact numbers yet. The research is still in its infancy. What we *do* know is that sitting for extended periods of time makes a mess of things. And we do know enough to make a difference.

The Solution

To avoid the dangers of sedentarism, you should first take a realistic look at your typical day. How active—and especially *inactive*—are you?

Then simply increase your movement throughout the day. Here are some specific solutions:

Break it up with a few minutes of moving. You can offset sedentary habits by getting up and moving around for a few minutes every hour—or, even better, every 30 minutes. Then do it again after another 30 to 60 minutes. Avoid spending big chunks of time sitting by squeezing in 5 to 10 minutes of activity whenever you can. Spend a few minutes on a treadmill or exercise bike, practice a couple Fit Quickies, do a few stretches, or curl some dumbbells. Walk to the far end of the office or your house to get a glass of water.

Stand up! Really, it's that easy. Standing commands a stronger metabolic response than either sitting or reclining. Your postural muscles spring into action with multiple stabilizing isometric contractions.

In studies of rats who were forced to be inactive, the leg muscles they used for standing lost more than 75 percent of their ability to remove harmful lipoproteins from the blood—almost immediately, as reported by Mark Hamilton and his team in 2003 in *The Journal of Physiology*. To see if the ill effects of sitting could have a rapid onset in humans, too, researchers recruited 14 young, fit, and thin volunteers. After just 24 hours of being sedentary, they recorded a 40 percent reduction in insulin's ability to uptake glucose in the subjects.

Get an adjustable-height workstation. This might not be possible for you, but it might not hurt to ask your company about this option as a tool for preventative wellness in the workplace. Employers looking to reduce "sick" time are wise to take a serious look at options such as this. If you work at home, you can rig your own setup.

If you must sit at a desk, spend some of that time sitting on a physioball. The destabilization effect of sitting on a large exercise ball keeps your core muscles lightly engaged.

Try for 5 to 10 minutes of activity every hour. That can mean a walk around the block, a climb up the stairs, 2 Fit Quickies, or a spin on the exercise bike. Stand rather than sit during phone calls. Take a short walk with every water break. Get creative in how you fit in nonsedentary bursts; every little bit helps!

NEAT—nonexercise activity thermogenesis (physiological process that produces heat) is the official term for the energy expenditure of daily activities such as standing, walking, talking, and sitting. None of these activities can be considered planned physical exercise of your daily life, yet with a little planning, they can have a dramatic impact. As a bonus, research has shown that including a little more NEAT in your life can burn up to an additional 350 calories a day.

If you work at home, it's even easier to meet your body's need for regular movement. Simply set a timer near your workstation or put an alert on your computer or smartphone for every 30, 45, or 60 minutes. When the alarm sounds, move your body. One of my favorite ways to do this is to pick a Fit Quickie or two. These are always fun and instantly invigorating.

Do Fitness Breaks Really Make a Difference?

In 2009, Dr. Peter Katzmarzyk and his colleagues at the Pennington Biomedical Research Center published a paper that examined the links between time spent sitting and mortality. The study included 17,000 people and found that time spent sitting was associated with increased risk of cardiovascular disease–related death.

But here's the kicker: the relationship between sitting time and mortality was *independent* of overall physical activity. In fact, subjects who sat the most were, give or take, 50 percent more likely to die during the follow-up period than individuals who sat the least. This was even after controlling for age, smoking, and physical activity levels, and independent of body weight.

So do those little breaks really make a difference? Yes! Research suggests that, in addition to the amount of sedentary time, the quality of that time may have an important health impact. To illustrate, in the Australian Diabetes, Obesity and Lifestyle Study, a total of 168 men and women aged 30 to 87 years wore an accelerometer to measure their bodily movement during all waking hours for 7 consecutive days. Using that data, researchers were able to quantify the amount of time participants spent being sedentary. This also told them how frequently the subjects punctuated sedentary activities with light activity, such as standing and walking to the restroom.

The data showed a direct correlation between the number of breaks taken from sitting behavior—especially more active breaks—and lower waist circumference, BMI, glucose tolerance, and blood lipids in the subjects. What's more, among nearly 9,000 Australians, for each additional hour of television a person sat and watched per day, his or her risk of dying rose by 11 percent, as established in 2008 by Genevieve Healy and her team at the University of Queensland.

Even if the total amount of sedentary and physical activity time were equal among individuals, those who took more frequent breaks while watching television or at work were less obese and had better metabolic health. And not much time and effort was involved. The breaks taken in this study were short—less than 5 minutes—and of low intensity, such as light walking or simply standing.

The big take-away here is this: all things being equal—age, gender, physical activity, body weight, smoking frequency, alcohol intake, age, and sex—the person who sits more is at a higher risk of disease and death than the person who sits less. I don't know about you, but this little nugget got me up of my chair, out the door to the deck, and on a 5-minute walking break.

Short or Long Workouts: Which Is Better?

Here's what the research says about many mini-workouts versus fewer longer workouts: pick the one you'll actually do. Recent studies concur that, when it comes to choosing between shorter workouts more often or fewer long workouts, the health benefits are about the same.

However, we now know it's essential to break up hours of sedentary inactivity with short sessions of activity. Punctuating sedentary stretches of time with motion—or simply standing up, for starters—is vital.

As a matter of fact, in one study, the short-bout exercisers experienced a greater reduction in BMI than the long-bout exercisers. One 10-week study compared the effects of long bouts of brisk walking among 47 women aged 38 through 61. They were randomly assigned to either three 10-minute walks per day (short bouts), one 30-minute walk per day (long bouts), or no training (control group). The intensity of the walking was consistent between the two groups, at 70 to 80 percent of maximal heart rate. Subjects agreed not to make changes to their diet.

At the end of the 1998 study conducted by M. Murphy and colleagues at the University of Ulster-Jordanstown in Northern Ireland, the sum of four skinfold site thicknesses decreased in both walking groups, but body mass and waist circumference decreased significantly only in short-bout walkers. Thus, short bouts of brisk walking resulted in similar improvements in fitness and were at least as effective in decreasing body fat as long bouts of the same total duration.

In study after study, no significant difference in results is reported between long-bout and short-bout exercise groups. Even if you have to break your activity, exercise, and workouts into shorter bites throughout the day, you benefit just as much as if you've done longer workouts in terms of improving your fitness, health, and body composition. This is great news when you want the benefits of exercise but can't find big chunks of time to fit it in. Plus, you gain the advantage of offsetting the damaging effects of big blocks of sedentary time.

In another study, marked improvement was shown in cardiorespiratory fitness and blood lipids when participants shifted out of sedentary mode into intermittently active mode. Fifteen women, whose age averaged 18.8 years old, were randomly assigned to control or stair-climbing groups. Stair-climbing progressively increased from one ascent a day in week 1 to 5 ascents a day in weeks 7 and 8. Training took place 5 days a week on a public-access staircase (199 steps), at a stepping rate of 90 steps a minute. Each ascent took about 2 minutes to complete. Subjects agreed not to change their diet or lifestyle over the experimental period.

The conclusion? The 2005 study, also from the University of Ulster-Jordanstown in Northern Ireland and conducted by C. A. Boreham and associates, confirmed that accumulating short bouts of stair-climbing activity throughout the day can favorably alter important cardiovascular risk factors in previously sedentary young women.

Those 30+ minutes of purposeful activity you should be doing each day can be chunked into shorter bites. That's a short walk, a spin on your exercise bike, or a few minutes of stair-climbing worked into your day. Then you can do those longer workouts and walks on the days when you have more time. You just took "I don't have time" off the "Why I don't exercise" list.

Fit Quickie #1

7 SECONDS TO A FLAT BELLY

Goal/results: Eliminate pooch, flatten your abdomen, strengthen your abdominal muscles, and improve your posture

Workout time: Less than 3 minutes

Equipment: None, other than a counter, chair, bar, or railing—anything will work—to use as an anchor point. You can even just touch a spot on the wall as an anchor. *Optional:* a 6- or 7-inch playground ball or pillow for the variation.

The Problem

I don't care who you are, belly pooch—that area right under your belt in front—is almost always an area of concern.

Whenever I teach this Fit Quickie, I always ask the question: "Does anyone *not* know what belly pooch is? Because if you don't, please present yourself ...." And without exception, almost before the words are out of my mouth, this question gets ripples of laughter.

We all know what belly pooch is. But what you may not know is what causes belly pooch. It's not necessarily what you think.

The Facts

One of the contributors to belly pooch is fat carried in the abdomen. Depending on your genetics, you might have a tendency to carry more or less body fat stores in your abdominal area.

But belly pooch also appears because the unchallenged abdominal muscles have relaxed and lost their girdling power. As your activity levels decline, those deep abdominal muscles become less firm than they were in your younger days, when you engaged in running, jumping, climbing, and playing for hours every day. Those activities challenged these muscles and made them better at their job of keeping your back, belly, and midsection intact.

The yogis have known this secret for centuries: this weakened muscle tone is compounded by the subsequent sinking of your internal organs lower into your abdominal cavity. That downward and outward pressure of your internal organs on your weak abdominal wall due to gravity's pull presses outward against the abdomen. Combined with reduced muscle tone in the muscles deep in the abdominal wall, you've got bulging belly pooch.

The full set of abdominal muscles—the rectus abdominis, the obliques, and the transversus abdominis—work together as a team, and it can be difficult, if not impossible, to isolate them completely. Together these muscles rotate and flex your trunk and pelvis. And when the entire set of muscles is engaged, it delivers stability to your spine. These muscles make it possible for you to perform a bending and twisting motion while supporting your spine. They are also important girdling muscles, forming a natural corset and holding your belly flat. This girdle protects you from both external abdominal pressure, such as a blow to the stomach, and intra-abdominal pressure, such as coughing or sneezing.

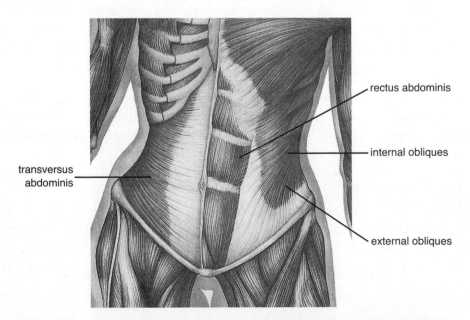

Your abdominal muscles are layered and work together to move and stabilize your body.

The abdominal muscle group includes the rectus abdominis, your "six-pack" muscle; the internal and external obliques, the "waist cinchers" that also work to flex, twist, and rotate your trunk; and the transversus abdominis, which provides deep girdling in the abdomen, flattening the abdominal wall and compressing the abdominal viscera.

This background information is key to understanding how Fit Quickie #1 provides you with a belly pooch solution. You're about to change your abdominal profile in the fastest, easiest way possible!

Queen of the Antipooch Prom

Of all the abdominal muscles, the transversus abdominis reigns supreme when it comes to protecting your lower abdominal cavity from internal as well as external pressure. That's why it tightens when you cough, grips when you sneeze, and flexes when you laugh. You also instinctively contract it when you anticipate a punch in the stomach. It's the deepest abdominal muscle and the most responsible for flattening your belly, coordinating with the obliques that work at keeping your waist cinched and tight.

The transversus abdominis muscle lies directly beneath the rectus abdominis muscle. It's the first in line of duty for keeping your natural corset doing its job. When you exhale, your transversus abdominis contracts and acts as an anchor and stabilizer for your other trunk muscles. Yet if you don't go out of your way to work this muscle, you lose your tight waist, your trunk stability, and your flat belly.

Check this out for yourself. Place your fingertips right below your beltline in front—yes, right on the "pooch" area. Now cough lightly or laugh. Feel that tightening beneath your fingertips? That's your abdominal muscles at work, holding your internal organs in place as pressure is created within your abdominal cavity.

Not Just for Looks

Your transversus abdominis muscle has several functions. One is to facilitate exhalation. As a matter of fact, when you want to blow out a breath quickly, like when you blow out candles on a birthday cake, this muscle scrambles into action to make it happen. During active expiration, the most important muscles are those of the abdominal wall (including the rectus abdominis, internal and external obliques, and transversus abdominis), which drive up intra-abdominal pressure when they contract. That pressure pushes up your diaphragm, raising pressure around your lungs and then within your alveoli, which drives out air. Everything works together to help you breathe and build that beautiful body.

Weakened abdominal muscles that result in belly pooch present more problems than just profile challenges. When your natural girdle starts to weaken, a whole series of problems can occur. You can develop back pain because the weakened abdominal wall results in excessive anterior pelvic tilt, tilting the top of your pelvis forward. (Remember this from the "Fit Quickie Fundamentals" chapter.) This creates a chain reaction of events that travels up your torso and spine as your body fights to maintain equilibrium and functional balance. The result? Faulty posture, back and neck pain, and alignment problems through your neck and head.

As this weakness persists and your natural girdle loses condition more, the pressure of the internal organs—now less firmly held in place—increases pressure on your pelvic floor, resulting in incontinence.

Worse, the transversus abdominis and the muscles of the pelvic floor are on the same neurological loop. Therefore, if the transversus abdominis isn't working properly, the other muscles won't function properly, either.

See how important strong abdominal muscles are? Let's get them in tip-top shape!

The Fit Quickie Fix

The great news is that you can target this deep abdominal muscle just like you would squeeze your fist. And that means you can train it to recover its girdling powers and get your natural corset back.

The transversus abdominis muscle responds quickly to isometric exercise, or strength training done in a static position rather than through a range of motion. You don't have to go anywhere or lift anything, which means you can sneak in Fit Quickie #1 anywhere, anytime, and no one will know but you. Talk about convenient!

Your transversus abdominis muscle works in concert with your diaphragm to expel breath from your lungs. A sharp exhalation immediately fires up your transversus abdominis muscle, engaging it and providing stability through your core muscles. By contracting your transversus abdominis, you create a back-protective splint with your spine. That's another reason to build your transversus abdominis strength with this Fit Quickie.

Here are a few of the benefits of including Fit Quickie #1 as part of your regular routine:

- It reverses abdominal muscle atrophy.

- It restores strength and tone to your abdominal wall.

- It flattens your abdomen.

- It improves your posture as you get your natural corset back in shape.

- It reverses symptoms of incontinence due to a weak abdominal wall and muscles of the pelvic floor.

How to Do It

Start by putting your body in optimal alignment for the Fit Quickie sequence. For Fit Quickie #1, it's simple.

Position

Here's your starting position:

1. Stand with your feet parallel and directly under your hip joints. Imagine you're standing on a pair of skis 4 or 5 inches apart.

2. Bend your knees slightly. Upright your spine so the weight of your ribs is stacked right over your hips. And as Miss H. taught me, lift the weight of your ribs vertically from your hips, creating more space in your torso. This immediately takes an inch off

your waist, and it decompresses your spine. It also brings focus and beauty and allows for more breath in your movements. If you're sunk into your lower body, you've squeezed out some breathing space. You want all the room for breath you can get.

3. Open your chest, with your shoulders back, and secure your position by engaging the muscles through your mid- and upper back to stabilize your upper-body posture. Have a sense of wrapping your shoulder blades securely around your rib cage in back.

4. Bring your pelvis into correct anatomical alignment. Remember, your lower back will have its natural curve. Contract lightly through your gluteals. Do not overgrip, try to flatten your back, or otherwise get carried away with lower body muscle activation. You want to create a solid foundation for your abdominal work without taking attention away from the isolations of your abdominal muscles. This is *anchored neutral*.

5. Press your crown, or the top of the head, to the ceiling. Keep your gaze forward and parallel to the ground so your lifted spine extends all the way up through your neck, keeping a sense of open energy all the way through the top of your head. You should now have a direct vertical line flowing from your ears through your shoulders to your hips.

Anchors

Place one hand on a contact point next to your body at about waist height. This can be a kitchen counter or bar, the back of a high chair, a dance bar, or anything else that will serve as a stabilizer. I've used my dance bar at home, a railing in the wait lounge of an airport, and even the back of a pickup truck between dives on a scuba adventure. Get creative! Remember, I said *anywhere*, *anytime* and I meant it.

Here are your anchor points for Fit Quickie #1:

- Your shoulder girdle stabilization from positioning

- Your feet on the floor

- Your hand on a stable surface

Isolate

In this exercise, your focus is on your transversus abdominis muscle. Remember, this is the deepest muscle in the abdominal muscle group, girdling the front of your abdomen and attaching to your ribs. You can find this muscle where it crosses in the "pooch" area easily, just a couple of inches below your belly button. To help you focus, place your free hand lightly on this area. You want to focus on the point of muscle activation. When you touch the place on your body where you want to focus, you establish a deeper brain-to-body connection.

 All the setup may seem detailed in the beginning, but you'll get the hang of it with just a little practice. After two or three times, you'll quickly and easily get into position and get started, posture perfect and ready to go.

Repetitions

Time for action! Let's start the reps.

Place your hand on your transversus abdominis area and blow out a breath rapidly, as if you were blowing out the candles on a cake. Feel it?

You're going to hook into that action for Fit Quickie #1, but in a more controlled fashion using your abdominals—led by your transversus abdominis— in an ever-increasing contraction to flatten and firm your lower abdominal area. It is possible to squeeze your transversus abdominis muscle very tight via isometric contraction. This is the skill you will develop with this exercise.

Here's how to do it:

1. Relax your abdomen, and take a deep breath.

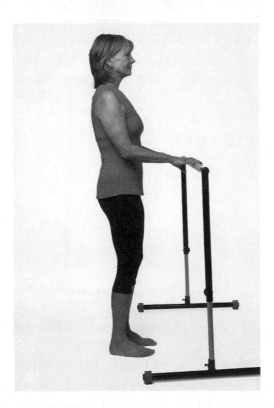

Keeping your body properly aligned, relax your abdomen and gently inhale. This is not the time to hold in your belly—that's next! For now, just let it go.

2. Exhale evenly and slowly for 7 seconds while consciously contracting your abdominal muscles by pulling them in. Maintain the rest of your anchored position throughout, and let your abs do the work!

3. While maintaining correct position and posture, and keeping your breath expelled and your abdominal muscles contracted to their max, continue to isometrically hold the contraction for 7 more seconds.

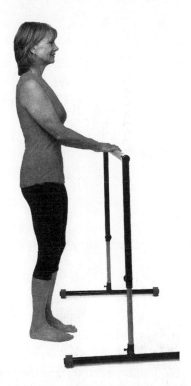

Exhale slowly and evenly, contracting your abdominal muscles by pulling those deep girdling muscles toward your spine. Then hold the abdominal muscles in flat and tight.

4. Gently relax your abdomen and your transversus abdominis muscle while you breathe back in for 7 counts. Be sure not to collapse the rest of your posture. Maintaining beautiful form trains your body to retain good functional form as you continue with the rest of your day after the exercise.

Reconnect with your position and anchors, and repeat for a total of 7 times.

Please note that if you find it difficult to hold your breath out after the exhale, or if this has been contraindicated for you for any reason, it's perfectly fine to breathe during the held contraction phase. Actually, doing so *increases* the isometric workload because you have to counterinstinctively hold your abdominal girdle tightly contracted against the expansion of the abdomen that comes naturally with an incoming breath.

It may take a few rounds or days of practice before you really feel your abdominal muscles working. If you can't find the deeper layers of muscle at first, keep working. You probably have reduced tone in your deep abdominal wall, which is part of the problem. This gives you a good reason to challenge your transversus abdominis and recover its power to flatten your belly, improve your posture, and bring better balance and stabilization to your core, which also protects your back.

To review, the sequence is as follows:

1. Relax and inhale.

2. Exhale for 7 seconds.

3. Isometrically hold your transversus abdominis for 7 seconds.

4. Relax and inhale.

Practice this exercise every day for the first week. Think of it as a belly boot camp. This will help you more quickly connect with the exercise and your transversus abdominis muscle. Then you can switch to four or five times a week or continue with more regular practice, if you like. In no time, you'll feel and see the difference in your abdominal profile.

Stretch

This is the only Fit Quickie that doesn't have a separate stretch. With this exercise, after each series of 7-count contractions and the following isometric hold, you relax your abdominal wall as you take a deep breath, essentially giving your abdominal muscles a release. The deep breath delivers all the stretch you need.

Variation: On the Floor

This variation challenges your transversus abdominis muscle in a slightly different way. It's also great for those who are unable to stand or sit. With this version, you add a new tool to your bag of body-shaping tricks.

In this version, you move to the floor. As you do this version in a lying-down position, you'll find that it's an exercise you're going to be able to fit in before you get out of bed in the morning. Talk about sneaking in exercise!

Position

Here's your position for the variation:

1. Lie on the floor on your back, with your knees bent, your feet flat on the floor, and your heels a comfortable distance from your rear end. Your toes should be straight ahead and your thighs should be parallel to each other.

2. Place a small hand towel, flat and two layers thick, under the natural curve in your lower back. This shouldn't be rolled up, take up too much space, or make you feel like your lower back is being pressed upward toward the ceiling. The purpose of the towel is to keep a curve in your back and add a small measure of resistance as you exhale and pull in your abdomen.

3. Let the backs of your shoulders drop into the floor behind you.

4. Let your spine lengthen as you feel your back release and extend from your tailbone up through the top of your head. You want your back to feel nice and long.

5. Place the ball between your knees to help you keep your knees, hips, and shoulders in proper alignment.

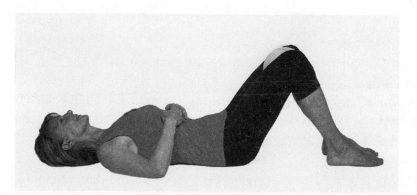

For this version, you complete all stages of the exercise on your back with your knees bent and your feet flat on the floor.

Anchor

Here are your anchor points:

- The playground ball between your knees, which brings your inner thighs into play as well—always a plus

- Your heels, hips, back, and the back of your head on the floor

 Let your body be heavy on the floor so you can put all your attention on your abdominal contractions.

- *Optional:* Place one hand on your belly as an anchor and focus point

Isolate

Isolation for this variation is the same as in the standing version.

Repetitions

This version has the same stages as the original:

1. Relax and inhale.

2. Exhale for 7 seconds.

3. Isometrically hold your transversus abdominis for 7 seconds.

4. Relax and inhale.

Note a few differences between the original Fit Quickie #1 and this version. In the variation, gravity is working in your favor. On your back, with your torso parallel to the floor, gravity helps pull your abdominal muscles in and toward the back of your body. Yet somehow this doesn't make it any easier—some people think it's even more challenging! One reason is because the rest of your body is relatively relaxed, and you can put all your attention on your transverses abdominis and other muscles of the abdominal wall.

This variation also gives you something to push against, if you use a small flat towel under your back. This can increase your concentration and connection with the exercise.

You'll become aware of the pelvis-tilting properties of your abdominal contractions in this version. The contraction of your abdominal muscles can actually tilt your pelvis by about 10 degrees. Any more than that, and you know you've activated your gluteals. Leave them out if it—we'll get to them later.

Remember, it's isolate and overload!

Common Errors

Beware of these common errors while you exercise:

- Don't allow your upper body to slump in the standing version.

- Don't create tension in your shoulders and face as you try to assist the abdominal contractions in both the standing and lying-down versions.

- Don't allow your pelvis to slip into an excessive anterior tilt.

Tips and Modifications

These tips and alternate ways to perform the exercise might help:

- Stay mindful of your position throughout, and reconnect with your correct posture between each round.

- Relax your face and keep your shoulders dropped down from your ears, even in the variation.

- As you progress, try imagining that you're pulling the fronts of your hip bones *toward* each other when you contract your abdominal muscles.

 You can easily do Fit Quickie #1 seated, whether you're at your office desk or in your car. Sometimes I do it while walking—if I've really got to sneak in some exercise in my day.

There you have it! Tuck this one into your routine four or five times a week, and say good-bye to belly pooch as you enjoy the improvements in your profile and your posture.

Fit Quickie #2
INNER THIGH SQUEEZE AND TEASE

Goal/results: Strengthen and shape the muscles of your inner thighs

Workout time: Less than 4 minutes

Equipment: Small 6- or 7-inch rubber playground ball or foam pillow; bar or counter as support for standing version

The Problem

Inner thigh challenged? You're not alone. The inner thigh is high on the out-of-shape list for so many of us. As discouraging as the state of your inner thighs may be, there is hope. Part of the problem is that these muscles just aren't challenged enough to keep some decent shape. Yet you can strengthen them to perform as good as new. It just takes some specific attention and a few simple strategies.

The inner thigh is also a zone where, based largely on your genetics, body fat is readily stored. And just like the belly pooch we talked about in Fit Quickie #1, an increase in the size of your inner thighs can be due to fat weight gain.

Remember, resistance exercise helps strengthen and shape muscles, but it doesn't spot reduce fat stores on your body. To create an overall leaner physique, you've got to eat healthier, too. With a healthy, low-fat diet, complemented by targeted muscle overload and regular cardiovascular exercise, you've got the winning ticket for changing the shape of your legs.

The Facts

The primary function of your inner thigh muscles group—officially known as the hip adductors—is hip adduction. Hip adduction occurs when you move your femur, the large thigh bone of your leg, in toward the midline of your body. These muscles also rotate your legs, flex your hips, and help stabilize your hip joints.

The adductor group includes five muscles: adductor magnus, adductor brevis, adductor longus, gracilis, and pectineus. You'd think with all those muscle-coordinating efforts, there'd be plenty of solid shape!

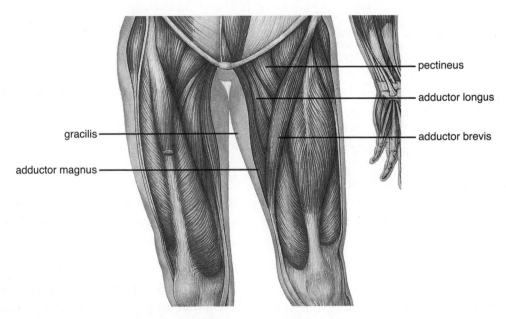

The hip adductor group is a working assembly of several muscles that run from your pubic bone to your inner thigh.

You use your adductor muscles with every step you take, as they work to keep your legs straight and keep you upright. However, these muscles are minimally challenged in most daily movements, as your other, larger, and stronger leg muscles tend to take over the workload. In other words, although they're assigned the job of stabilization, the muscles of the inner thighs can more easily just go along for the ride. And if you simply aren't moving around much, they get even weaker, compounding the problem.

Most people don't think of the inner thigh muscles as core muscles, but all the leg adductor muscles originate on the pelvic bone and attach at intervals along the length of the femur, the large bone in your upper leg. This interval-attachment design provides power and stability for your hip joints and femurs, especially when you're standing on one leg.

Multijoint exercises for the lower body, such as squats, plies, and lunges, involve the adductors and are part of a solid overall conditioning program. These exercises work on shaping your legs as a whole. They are compound movements that use your inner thighs to stabilize the rest of your body, and you should include them in your exercise rotation. (For a super shaper squat exercise, see Fit Quickie #12, a personal favorite.)

Depending on the design of the exercise, the stronger muscles of the legs may work together to take on a big chunk of the work, especially if the exercises also call on the quadriceps and hamstrings, the muscles that make up the front and back of the upper legs, respectively. This can lead to underdevelopment of the adductor group. It's no wonder they can become weak. Some isolation work is definitely in order.

The Fit Quickie Fix

Conditioned inner thigh muscles create shapely legs, restore a power and grace to your stride, help improve your posture, aid in knee joint stabilization, and just plain help build physical beauty and confidence.

As noted earlier, you need a small playground ball for this exercise. A piece of foam rubber or a small foam pillow also works, but as a second choice. Something with strong resiliency gives you a better thigh challenge for this exercise, and the playground ball does this best. It has "fight back" qualities that deliver better resistance.

How to Do It

You can practice this exercise in a standing or seated position. The standing version steps up the challenge to your overall body. It gets you up on your feet, where I want you as often as possible. You'll feel the activation not only in your inner thigh muscles, but also in the muscles in the fronts of your thighs, your quadriceps, as you invite them into the action. Yet due to the unique positioning of Fit Quickie #2, you still shine the bigger spotlight on the muscles of your inner thighs. The trick is to be aware of your quadriceps working without letting them take over the show.

The standing version gets you up on your feet, challenging more muscles, so it's the bigger calorie-burner of the two. At the same time, the seated version leaves no question as to whether you've "isolated and overloaded" those leg adductors. Pick your favorite variation and alternate them between your workout sessions, or as you do two sets of the exercise each time, complete one set of each.

I set up the standing version first and then show you how to modify for the seated version.

Position

Here's how to get into position for the standing version:

1. Stand with your feet parallel, about 5 inches apart.

2. Place the ball between your thighs, slightly above your knees, and grasp it firmly.

3. Stand tall, lift the weight of your ribs off your hips, and extend the top of your head to the ceiling.

4. Bring your spine into neutral position, with the natural curves in your back keeping their integrity, gluteals active, and with a neat vertical line from your ears through your shoulders and through your hips. Engage your abdominal muscles to help line things up. Remember, your abdominal muscles will remain as active stabilizers throughout the exercise.

5. Your chest should be open, and your shoulder blades anchored on your rib cage in back, stabilizing your upper body. Elegance, confidence, and beautiful intention of movement are now yours.

6. Keeping a firm grasp on the ball and maintaining your upper-body position, place your hand lightly on a bar, chair, or counter to assist with posture. Bend your knees to gently lower yourself straight down an inch or two—no leaning backward or forward. Keep your heels on the floor. This isn't a deep knee bend. Bend your knees just enough to create a deeper workload through your lower body.

7. In this slightly bent-knee position, pull in your abdominal wall and grip your glutes slightly to regain anchored neutral position. Your body will want to adapt to the balance challenge by leaning your upper body forward and letting your tail lift in back, pitching your pelvis into excessive anterior tilt. However, your mission is to maintain your spinal alignment and position. This is key to creating safer exercise and more functional, beautiful posture. To do so, you'll notice your abdominal muscles need to fire up a little more, and your gluteal muscles also jump into the game a bit. That's how it should be, so allow it to happen, but only to keep your pelvis level and your spine in proper position as you lower.

8. In bent-knee position, check again that you've maintained the integrity of your upper-body alignment before proceeding. There should still be a direct line through your ears, shoulders, and hips. Level your chin, and avoid looking down because it starts to collapse your posture—we can't have that! Keep your gaze forward.

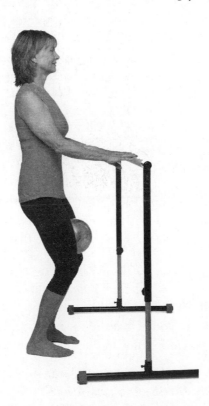

Lower only slightly so you don't fire up the muscles on the fronts of your thighs too much.
Concentrate on squeezing the ball between your thighs.

Anchors

Here are your anchor points:

- Your feet on the floor

- Your thighs gripping the ball

- Your shoulder blades wrapped securely against your rib cage in back

- Your hand on the bar or chair

- Your abdominals and glutes actively maintaining anchored neutral position

Isolate

Gripping the playground ball as a point of anchor isolates your inner thigh muscles. You'll feel them fire up right away, and combined with the activation of your gluteals and quadriceps from your anchored pelvis and your slightly bent knee position, you'll quickly become aware of isometric load throughout your lower body. Keep the ball firmly gripped, and you're ready for repetitions.

Repetitions

Here's the breakdown for Fit Quickie #2:

1. Squeeze your knees toward each other, pressing the ball for a slow initial count of 10 squeezes. This is the initial squeeze. Don't be too quick to let go of the squeeze. Spend more of each repetition in the squeeze than the release.

2. Now for the tease phase: do 2 squeezes followed by a hold squeeze for 10 rounds. The count goes like this: squeeze, squeeze, squeeze and hold, squeeze, squeeze, squeeze and hold. Hold the squeeze during the third section so you have actually 2 counts of squeeze. Notice that the squeeze count outnumbers the release counts. That's so you spend more time in the muscle contraction, building the workload.

3. Finish with 20 rapid squeezes, like this: squeeze, squeeze, squeeze, ….

4. Take a short rest before repeating the entire sequence. Pull out of your bent knees to straightened legs for a brief break as needed.

 Although the inner thigh muscles are notoriously tough to target, with Fit Quickie #2, I guarantee you'll find those muscles fast. You'll love the results—inner thighs that are tighter in appearance and firmer in feel.

Variation: Seated

If knee or ankle issues impair your ability to do Fit Quickie #2 standing, you can modify the exercise by practicing in a seated position.

Position

Here's how to get into position:

1. Sit on a firm chair or bench, inching forward on the chair so your knees extend 10 to 12 inches beyond the edge of the seat. You should have a 90-degree bend in your knees, with your feet flat on the floor, directly beneath your bent knees.

2. Sit upright on your "sitz" bones, the common name for the *ischial tuberosity* and the lowest of the three major bones that make up the pelvis. It's the part of your pelvis that takes your weight when you sit.

3. Sit away from the chair back so you can create an upright spine and create correct alignment, as you would in the standing version, anchoring your shoulder blades securely on your back, your abdominals engaged, and your spine upright.

4. Place the ball between your knees, slightly above your knees toward your body on your inner thigh.

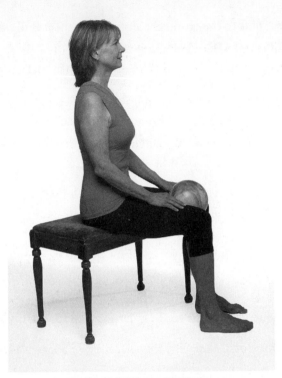

Fit Quickie #2, seated variation.

Anchors

Here are your anchor points:

- Your seat on the chair

- Your feet on the floor

- Your shoulder blades wrapped securely against your rib cage in back

- Your hand placed lightly on a desk, an armchair, or your thighs or waist

- The ball grasped between your knees, the contact point you'll be leveraging your work against

Isolate

Gently gripping the ball as a point of anchor isolates your inner thigh muscles. You'll notice right away how easy it is to find the appropriate muscles with this simple step.

Repetitions

Here's the breakdown for Fit Quickie #2, seated version (these are the same steps as for the standing version):

1. Squeeze your knees toward each other, pressing the ball for a slow initial count of 10 squeezes. This is the initial squeeze.

2. Now for the tease phase: do 2 squeezes followed by a hold squeeze for 10 rounds. The count goes like this: squeeze, squeeze, squeeze and hold, squeeze, squeeze, squeeze and hold. Hold the squeeze during the third section so you have actually 2 counts of squeeze. Notice that the squeeze count outnumbers the release counts. That's so you spend more time in the muscle contraction, building the workload.

3. Finish with 20 rapid squeezes, like this: squeeze, squeeze, squeeze, ….

4. Take a short rest before repeating the entire sequence.

Stretch

An important rule of muscle isolation work is to stretch the muscles you've isolated and worked immediately after the workload. This helps you maintain flexibility in the targeted muscles and joints.

Move to the floor for the stretch that follows the work portion Fit Quickie #2:

1. Sit in a straddle position with your legs extended in front of you in a wide V, with your heels on the floor and your toes to the ceiling.

2. Upright your spine and sit high on your sitz bones. You want that same beautiful posture you built in the standing and seated positions. Keep your back long and your spine lifted.

3. Place your hands shoulder width apart on the floor in front of you. If you can't reach the floor, either use a yoga block or place your hands on the tops of your thighs. The width of your straddle isn't important—the correct positioning and the stretch are. If you're not able to sit correctly in the straddle position, place a small pillow or a folded towel under your seat to create an elevator.

4. Keeping your back long and lifted, press your chest forward, keeping your toes toward the ceiling and your legs straight although not locked. Imagine you have a magnet on your chest pulling you forward. Extend your tailbone with a gentle lift toward the wall behind you, and press forward $\frac{1}{2}$ inch with your collarbone. This may be all you need to do to feel the stretch through your inner thighs, hips, and hamstrings, depending on your anatomy and flexibility. As with all stretches, it's not important how far you go; the stretch in the muscle is more important.

5. Breathe deeply and hold this stretch for 20 to 30 seconds; release and repeat.

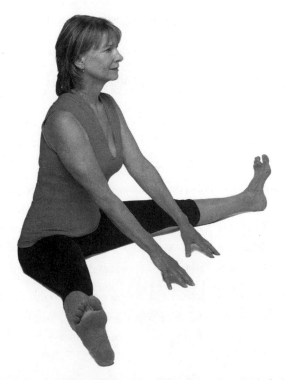

Gently press forward with your chest into the stretch. The important part is feeling the stretch, not seeing how far you can go.

Common Errors

Beware of these common errors while you exercise:

- In both variations, don't let go of your grip on the ball, allowing yourself to check out of the workload. Go for the gusto! The harder the workload here, the more you get out of fewer repetitions.

- In the standing version, don't neglect to pay attention to correct upper-body posture when lowering your body. Your body will want to check out of the work of stabilizing your abdominal muscles, your back muscles, and gluteal muscles. Always remain mindful of elegant, lifted, correct, and safe anatomical alignment.

Tips and Modifications

These tips and alternate ways to perform the exercise might help:

- Do your first set seated and your second set standing. This allows your knees to warm up and the rest of your body to scramble into readiness for the standing challenge. Of course, you can do both sets seated or standing.

- Minimize the rebound. In other words, keep the release that comes on the end of each squeeze small. Try to stay connected to working your muscles with short intervals of release.

- Other than your anchor points and the stabilization and supporting roles of your abdominals, back, quadriceps, and gluteal muscles, keep the rest of your body out of the action. You'll involve the rest of your body only as much as is needed to create good position, connect with your anchor points, and maintain the proper alignment you set up in the positioning phase.

- As another variation, you can try this lying on your back on the floor, with the ball between your knees and your feet flat on the floor and your knees bent at 90 degrees.

This Fit Quickie is so quick, convenient, and fun, you might be compelled to sneak it in more frequently than you need. But be careful not to overdo it. Remember, your muscles need to be not only challenged but also brought into balance. The leg adductors, challenged with Fit Quickie #2, need to be functionally complemented with a strong gluteus medius, which helps moderate leg adduction. Be sure to balance Fit Quickie #2 with exercises targeting your gluteus medius and other important muscles of your lower extremities. Fit Quickies #4, #5, and #12 are good for this.

Fit Quickie #3
TRICEPS TRIPLE PLAY

> **Goal/results:** Shape and strengthen the upper back of your arms
>
> **Workout time:** 5 minutes
>
> **Equipment:** Dumbbell, starting with 1 pound and working your way up to 3 or 5 pounds, and a sturdy platform upon which to kneel, such as a window seat, hearth, piano bench, or gym bench

The Problem

The triceps. That arm jiggle. Why is this area of the arm such a universal concern?

Although your daily activities and even many exercises utilize the triceps muscle, it's not nearly enough to give it a challenge that's going to make a difference in its shape. And unless you place a strong workload of demand on your triceps, it'll continue to lose size and shape. To make matters worse, body fat accumulates on the backs of the arms—especially for women.

Most people's triceps muscle is relatively weak. If yours is, you'll notice it right away when you isolate this muscle, just as you're about to do in Fit Quickie #3.

The Facts

The triceps is the muscle most responsible for giving shape to your arms. Sculpted triceps make your upper arms look more slender.

The triceps is challenging to work yet easy to isolate and overload, so results come quickly. Once you start working this muscle with Fit Quickie #3 and observe the results, you'll find triceps work to be a rewarding favorite.

The Fit Quickie Fix

Remember, Fit Quickies are research driven. I wanted to find the best movement principles for targeting those shape- and strength-challenged hot spots. Fit Quickie #3 is no exception. In a nonbiased study designed to determine which exercises are most effective and efficient for targeting the triceps, the triceps–kickback exercise, upon which Fit Quickie #3 is based, came out in the top two. I made the kickback even better by layering variations of movement within the exercise, in a specific sequence, to challenge the triceps in a unique, fast-acting way.

All muscles pull. Understanding how the triceps works helps you visualize and practice this Fit Quickie most effectively. The triceps muscle has three heads and three pulling jobs:

- It extends your arm by pulling it straight at the elbow.

- It works in concert with the latissimus dorsi muscle in the back to pull your arm closer to your body.

- It coordinates with the back of your shoulder to extend your arm behind you.

Unless you're rowing with oars, performing the challenging holds of a gymnast, or kneading bread on a regular basis, you can see why this muscle is a problem area for many of us.

I designed Fit Quickie #3 to target all three of these heads and functions of the triceps muscle in one tidy, fast exercise.

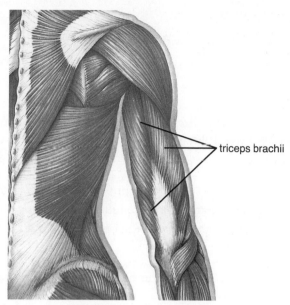

triceps brachii

The triceps is called a three-headed muscle because it contains three bundles of muscles, each with a different point of origin, that join at the elbow.

How to Do It

Precision with this exercise makes all the difference. You may be surprised at how quickly you feel your triceps working to fatigue. In fact, you might only be able to do a few repetitions at first. What's important is challenging your muscle, not how many reps you can do.

 If you're just starting out, try this exercise with no additional weight—I assure you it'll be challenging enough. When applying correct form to this exercise, you'll be astonished at how little weight you need to create the powerful workload you're looking for. If you're doing Fit Quickie #3 correctly, it doesn't take a whole lot of weight to get a good triceps workout.

Position

Here's your starting position, beginning with your right arm:

1. Kneel on the platform with your left knee.

2. Place your left hand on the platform directly beneath your left shoulder. Keep your right foot on the floor to stabilize the workload. This should put you in a position where your upper back and shoulders will probably be slightly higher off the platform than your hips.

3. Your neck should be in alignment with your spine. Imagine a straight line from your tail through your neck and extending through the top of your head. Remember all you learned about correct alignment of the upper body in Fit Quickies #1 and #2, and apply it to this horizontal position.

4. Keep your gaze slightly forward of your hand on the platform without lifting your head or letting it turn to the side.

5. Release your shoulders down and away from your ears. Keep your chest open and your shoulders back, your shoulder blades anchored on your rib cage in back, and your hips square to the floor and the platform. Your body will want to check out of the workload by trying to rotate your upper body open to the side of the arm you're working, so be sure to keep your start position straight and strong.

If you can't continue the repetitions in correct form, stop, let your arm extend toward the floor, roll your shoulder to release it, and bring your arm back up into position to reset your form. Then continue the exercise. If you can't complete all repetitions in correct alignment at first, that's fine. You'll work your way up as you get stronger. Fewer repetitions done with good form is far better than more repetitions without correct position.

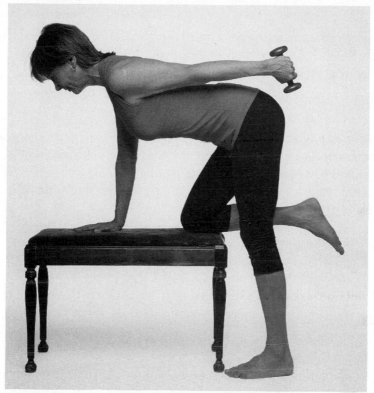

Extend your arm into a straight line from your wrist to your shoulder, with your arm close to your body.

Anchors

Here are your anchor points:

- Your knee on the platform

- Your hand on the platform

- Your foot on the floor

- The muscles and the middle of your back stabilized and keeping your chest open

- The shoulders anchored in position

- Your abdominals pulled in and isometrically engaged to stabilize your core

Isolate

To isolate your triceps muscle, with your arm straight and close to your body, raise your right arm directly behind you to or slightly above your hip. The idea is to get your right arm as close to parallel to the floor as possible. Again, keep your arm close to your body, your palm facing inward toward, and your body and your shoulders square.

 If you're holding a dumbbell, maintain a gentle hold on it and keep your wrist straight. Bringing your arm to this position with a straight elbow joint makes you aware of your triceps muscle jumping into action right away, and that's what you want. This is a signal that you've isolated your triceps muscle.

Repetitions

The repetitions follow a sequence of six different combinations. These layer the workload to give you the most challenge in the shortest amount of time.

Here's the breakdown for Fit Quickie #3:

1. In the starting position, with your arm raised straight to your side to above hip level, squeeze your arm even closer to your body in a tiny muscle-activating action. Your arm might barely move an inch, and it'll seem almost like an isometric squeeze with a bit of movement to keep things interesting. Here's the pattern: pull in, squeeze, hold; pull in, squeeze, hold. Each pull in, squeeze, and hold pattern takes a total of 2 seconds. Remember to keep your arm close to your body, with your elbow straight.

2. This adds another small move to step 1. You're going to pull in for 2 counts, lift your arm directly behind you, and hold. The lift to the back is also a small move, but it's deep in the triceps muscle. Your arm stays straight. Try it: pull in, pull in, lift, and hold; pull in, pull in, lift, and hold. The lift is small; it can be measured in inches. Each repetition of this pattern also takes about 2 seconds.

3. Now while continuing to keep your right arm straight and close to your body, lift your arm to the back for 8 counts. Again, the range of motion is small, and the repetition tempo is about 1 per second.

4. Keeping your arm lifted to the back, bend your elbow only slightly and then extend it straight for 8, again on a count of 1 per second. The bend should be small so you minimize the rebound from the contraction and straighten your arm. You'll feel this deep in your triceps muscles.

5. Next is a brief resetting of the position. Let your right arm drop so your hand extends toward the floor, roll your right shoulder, reset the square of your shoulders and the anchor of your shoulder blades with your back muscles, anchor your abdominals, and come back up to position for the final steps.

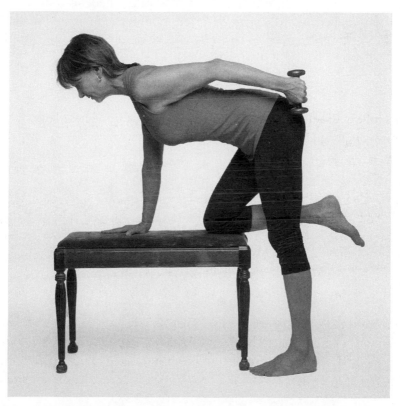

Bend your elbow a small amount and then put all the gusto you have into straightening your arm again. You'll feel this right away.

6. Keeping your elbow in place, and without letting it drop an inch, bend your elbow into a 90-degree bend and then straighten it into the start position. Take 1 second to bend and 1 second to straighten. Remember to straighten your arm all the way! Do this for 8 repetitions.

7. Now to finish off the workload of all three heads of your triceps. As you keep your arm close to your body, with your elbow straight and the back of your shoulder and arm working in concert, do 8 repetitions of the straight arm lifts.

Repeat the exercise sequences on your left arm. You want to kneel on your right knee with your right hand on the bench or platform, your left foot on the floor, and work the triceps in your left arm.

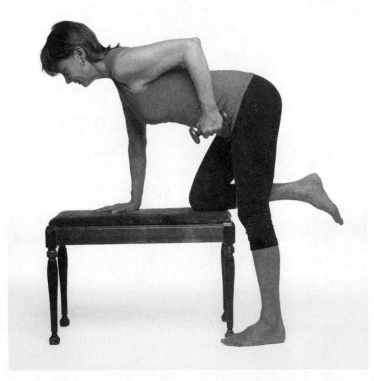

It's tempting to keep your elbow from straightening all the way when you bring it back up. Concentrate and make it happen.

Stretch

When you're finished with both arms, it's time to stretch your triceps:

1. Put your weights down and, sitting or standing, extend your right arm straight past your ear toward the ceiling.

2. Bending your right elbow, drop and reach your right hand down to the back of your neck or lower.

3. Bring your left hand up to grasp your right elbow, and gently pull on your right elbow. You'll feel the intense stretch down your triceps and down the side of your torso as well. Hold for 20 to 30 seconds and repeat with your other arm.

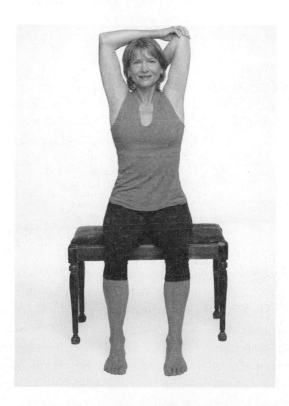

Concentrate on your strong upper-body posture as you stretch your triceps. Keep both shoulders down from your ears, even while you're reaching overhead, to help maintain integrity of your shoulder joints.

Common Errors

Beware of these common errors while you exercise:

- Be sure to straighten your arm completely when directed to do so, without locking or hyperextending your joint. Check your position in a mirror, if you can. Even if you think your arm is straight at the elbow, it might be slightly bent. Pushing yourself to really extend-extend-extend your arm straighter makes a big difference. I catch myself with a not-so-straight arm all the time and have to remind myself to straighten it. If you can't extend your arm straight, it may be that you're using too much resistance and need to use a lighter weight.

- Be sure to bring your working arm up as close to parallel to the floor as possible. The greatest resistance occurs at full extension of your arm when the resistance travels parallel to gravity. If you can't get your arm into parallel position, try it with a lighter weight.

- Don't allow your torso to rotate in the direction of your working arm. Your stronger shoulder and back muscles will want to take over the workload and give your triceps a break. That's nice of them, but it's not what you want here. You want to challenge your triceps! Keep your chest square to the floor, and let your arm do the work.

Tips and Modifications

These tips and alternate ways to perform the exercise might help:

- You can do this exercise in a standing lunge position if you're unable to kneel. Step your left foot forward, and bend your knee into a partial lunge position, with your right leg extended behind you. Fold forward at your hips, and rest your left hand on your left thigh. This becomes your "bench." Keep your shoulders square to the floor; somehow this lunge-position version makes it easier to twist your torso and check out of the primary workload. It also can make it more difficult to move your working arm into parallel due to the position your upper body is in. For these reasons, use the kneeling version whenever possible.

• If you're thinking, *I'll just start with a 5-pound dumbbell so I get the most out of the exercise*, guess again! This sequence is tough, and if you can get through it the first time with a 5-pound weight, I guarantee you're not straightening your arm, or you're rotating your upper body, your arm isn't in parallel, or all three. Form is more important here than repetitions, and you want to do fewer repetitions well than do a whole bunch of them of lesser quality. For your first time out, you don't have to hold a weight at all, and I guarantee you will feel it. Even as I've worked my way up from lower to higher weight, I can do this exercise with no weight and, by focusing on form and squeeze, still feel it. The shaping you're after is a result of the work you do, so do the work!

If you're new to what it feels like to really isolate and overload your muscles, you'll become familiar with that feeling quite quickly with Fit Quickie #3. Once you start to see the effects of this exercise, you'll be hooked.

Fit Quickie #4
GORGEOUS GLUTES AND HAMSTRINGS

> **Goal/results:** Shape, lift, and strengthen your gluteal muscles, a.k.a. your rear end
>
> **Workout time:** 3 minutes
>
> **Equipment:** 12×12-inch piece of 1-inch foam padding, rolled; a 6- or 7-inch playground ball

The Problem

If you're on a quest to get some shape in your posterior, you're not alone. The gluteals, one of the largest muscle groups in your body, are also one of the biggest reasons people exercise. If a nice, curvaceous rear is on your body-shaping wish list, you need muscle and you need no-nonsense strategies to counter the effects of gravity that may be moving things south.

Not only that, but weak, underdeveloped gluteal muscles contribute to back pain. Your glutes form a foundation of support for your upper body, and when that foundation is weak, the scaffold starts to crumble.

Most people have weak gluteal muscles. For one, we sit on them—a lot—and they've become overstretched and unconditioned. Sound familiar? The glutes get lazy and, unless your gluteal muscles are already strong, they're all too willing to let your lower back and hamstrings do the work.

Even if you do exercises specifically for your gluteals, you might be doing them wrong. I've often observed people inadvertently transfer the heavy lifting to their lower back—which has been carrying the workload anyway. The poor glutes never get a chance to show their stuff or reap the rewards of a job well done. It's time to fix that.

The Facts

Firmed, conditioned gluteals don't just look great; they're also important core muscles that provide solid stability to your back and lower torso. They also help ensure great posture and prevent back pain. And finally, being among the largest muscles on the body, getting them fired up during your workouts means engaging lots of muscle fibers, which translates into burning lots of calories. Conditioned gluteals also deliver a bounce to your step. There's no feeling quite like having your rear in gear.

 Your gluteals include three main muscles: the maximus, the largest portion of your backside; the medius, the pork-chop-shape muscle near the top of your hips; and the minimus, which is tucked neatly beneath the other two gluteal muscles. Fit Quickie #4 hits all three.

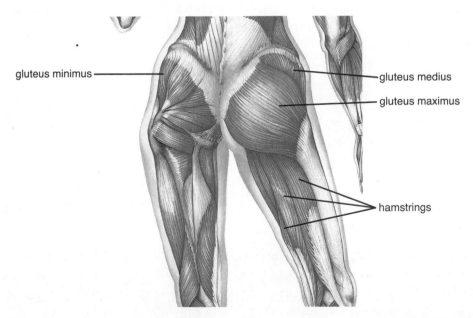

gluteus minimus

gluteus medius

gluteus maximus

hamstrings

Your gluteal muscles hitch up with your hamstrings in Fit Quickie #4 to build a strong and beautiful backside.

The Fit Quickie Fix

Although the shape of your backside and how easily you can develop muscles is largely due to genetics, the rest is influenced by exercise, posture, and nutrition—all details you can control. You can make a dramatic difference back there, and Fit Quickie #4 gives you the tools to do just that. I know you're going to love this move.

On a personal note, I've always had a flatter shape through my posterior. Yet thanks to Fit Quickies #4, #5, #8, #9, and #12, working together in concert, I've got an entirely reshaped profile back there.

I designed Fit Quickie #4 based on some very important research recently completed by the American Council on Exercise. Their goal was to get to the bottom (sorry!) of the most effective exercise for your rear end. This research compared eight exercises for the hamstrings and gluteals to determine which provided the strongest muscle fiber activation, measured using electromyography (EMG). The quadruped hip extension exercise, upon which Fit Quickie #4 is based, came up the winner for both muscles.

Electromyography, or EMG, is a technique for recording and evaluating the electrical activity produced by skeletal muscles. Through the use of the electromyograph, we can determine which movements get the most muscle fibers engaged. This helps determine which exercises may be most effective for any particular muscle or group of muscles.

You know you can count on me for some extra *umph* and challenge to isolation work. I've taken it a step further in this Fit Quickie by adding the extra workload of the hamstring squeeze.

For the squeeze, all you need is a small piece of foam padding about 1 inch thick and 12 inches square. You'll use this to intensify the isolation of the muscles you're targeting along the back of your thigh and into your seat, your hamstrings, and your gluteals. You'll sandwich the foam behind your knee between your hamstring and the top of your calf.

Here's the secret of the squeeze: as you grip the foam, you isolate and contract the hamstring muscle on the back of your thigh. When combined with the contraction of your gluteals to lift your leg into the repetitions, your hamstring and gluteals quickly scramble at their point of tie-in right at the base of your rear end and top of your thigh in back. This translates into an upward push of your hamstrings into your contracting glutes, bringing you the best of both worlds—the ultimate seat-shaping exercise. Once you feel this happen, you know you're on to something good.

How to Do It

You can place emphasis on different gluteal muscles depending on how you rotate your working leg at your hip. This shifting in focus is built into Fit Quickie #4, creating a comprehensive exercise for your glutes.

Position

Here's your starting position:

1. Begin on your hands and knees on the floor. Your hands should be right under your shoulders, and your knees directly beneath your hips. Think "on all fours," and you're there.

2. Pull in your abdominals and tilt the top of your pelvis slightly back as you gently tuck your tailbone. As soon as you begin to work, your pelvis will want to sneak into an anterior tilt and sway your lower back to make the job easier. You don't want that. Starting out with preemptive positioning aligned with your muscles activated helps keep your spine in anchored neutral position.

3. Square your hips to the floor and keep them this way throughout the exercise. Imagine you have headlights on your hip bones shining straight onto the floor to help keep correct position. As you progress, your gluteals will want to get some relief from the workload and encourage you to open your hip outward to make it easier. Remember those headlights, and maintain correct position.

These positioning elements together provide a stable platform for the exercise and increase the focus of the workload just where you want it, through your hamstrings and continuing up into your gluteals.

4. Keep a long line through your spine to your neck and out the top of your head. Avoid letting your head droop or lifting your head to look up, both of which may create tension through your shoulders. At the same time, keep your shoulders down from your ears and your chest open by staying strong in your upper and middle back. Your shoulder blades anchored on your rib cage in back help stabilize your upper body.

Anchors

Here are your anchor points:

- Your knees on the floor

- Your hands on the floor

- Your abdominals firmly contracted

- Your shoulder blades locked on your rib cage in back

Isolate

To isolate your hamstrings and gluteals, you begin by grasping the piece of rolled foam behind your knee. If you start with the workload on your right leg, keep your left knee on the floor and sandwich the foam behind your right knee. This fires up your hamstrings immediately.

Keep the position elements in place with the top of your pelvis tilted slightly back and your abdominal wall pulled in. Raise your right knee with the foam tucked in directly behind you. You might find that you don't get your knee that high off the ground, but that's okay. It's important not to let your lower back sway to let the top of your pelvis pop forward toward the floor beneath you. The isolation of your hamstrings and gluteals is the priority here, not how high you can get your knee; raise your knee only until you feel your hamstring catch at the lower part of your seat. That "catch" is where your contracted hamstring and gluteals are scrambling at their point of tie-in. This is your position.

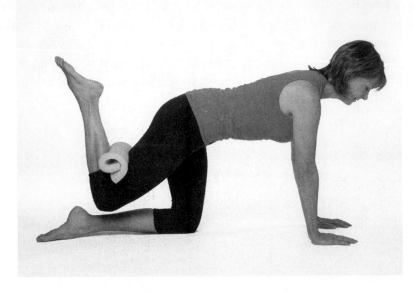

Grasping the foam pad and lifting your knee off the floor immediately fires up your hamstring and gluteal muscles.

Repetitions

Repetitions for this exercise follow seven different combinations, layering the workload to give you the most challenge in the shortest amount of time:

1. Squeeze and release the piece of foam behind your right knee for 8 slow counts, about 1 squeeze per second. Keep the release tiny so you stay in the muscle contraction.

2. Hold the foam pad grasped into the squeeze, and with the foot of your right leg relaxed, press the toes of that foot toward the ceiling by pulling from your gluteals. Be mindful of pulling with your glutes rather than just kicking your foot upward. Work it as hard as you can in a small range of motion for 8 counts. Each lift and hold should take about 1 second.

3. Deliberately bring your knee down to the floor and it back up again, consciously pulling from your gluteals. Each move of your knee toward the floor and back up should take about 2 seconds—down for 1 and up for 1. Complete 8 repetitions.

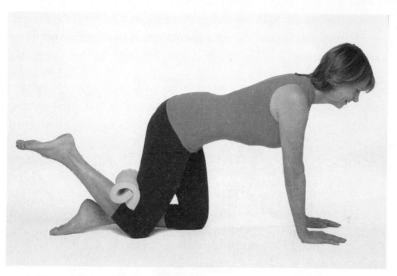

Always bring mental focus to the muscles you're targeting. In this case, pull from your glutes to lift your leg.

4. Move back into your starting position with your knee lifted off the floor and your toe to the ceiling. Complete 20 rapid presses of your toe toward the ceiling, using a small range of motion and staying mindful of keeping your pelvis anchored, your tail slightly tucked under, and your abdominals engaged. Complete about 2 tiny lifts a second.

Don't be surprised if you notice your left leg—the leg on the floor—experiencing a workload of its own. Along with your abdominals, it's braced to help stabilize you.

5. Staying in control, bring your knee down and let go of the foam. Extend your right leg straight out behind you on the floor. Again, keep your hips squared, the headlights on your hips shining forward, your abdominals in, and your pelvis slightly tucked. Now raise your leg up behind you with your foot gently flexed. Bring it up as high as you can without letting go of your proper hip pelvic position. Again, height is not important here. Keeping your leg straight, press your heel to the wall behind you, keeping your leg close in line with the midline of your body. At the top of the move, turn the toes of your right foot toward the wall on your right. You'll

feel a slight opening of your hip with this move as you rotate your leg and further engage your gluteus medius. All your glutes are in play here; you've just shifted the target zone somewhat.

Begin with 8 slow repetitions at the top of the lift. Keep the range of motion small, minimizing rebound and working deep in the muscle. Each lift should take about 1 second.

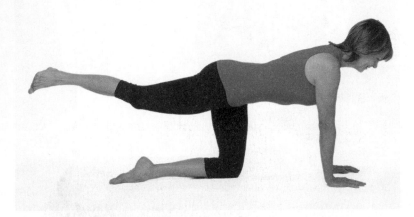

Rotate your working leg outward to shift the challenge on your gluteals. Be sure to keep your abdominals fired up and maintain proper shoulder position.

6. Squeeze and tease—lift, lift, lift, and hold your extended leg for 5 sets. Each lift, lift, lift, and hold should take about 2 seconds total.

7. Keeping your leg extended straight and still with your toes rotated out, complete 20 quick, small lifts. Stay mindful of keeping your abdominal and hip position.

Repeat steps 1 through 5 on your left leg. Then it's time to stretch.

Stretch

Now for a rewarding stretch:

1. Lie on your back with your knees bent and your feet flat on the floor. Cross your right knee over your left knee.

2. Keeping your back lengthened, retaining its natural curve on the floor and your shoulders pulled down and away from your ears, lift your feet off the floor, bringing your knees directly toward the center of your chest as you fold your legs toward you.

3. Reach toward your knees with your hands, and gently pull them closer toward your chest to increase the stretch in your hips. You'll feel this in your gluteals as well as in your lower back. Hold for 20 to 30 seconds before gently releasing and repeating on your other leg.

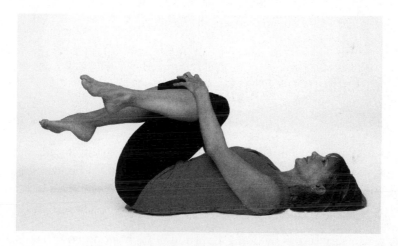

Allow your shoulders to drop back into the floor, and enjoy the release of the muscles in your hips as they relax into the stretch.

You'll probably feel the results of Fit Quickie #4 the next day. You'll also notice quite quickly how much more solid and better shaped you start to feel throughout your lower body.

Common Errors

Beware of these common errors while you exercise:

- Don't let go of your alignment through your pelvis and lower back—don't allow your back to sway or let your body check out of the workload. Repeatedly reconnect with the position principles, and avoid being competitive about how high you get your leg. It's not important how high you can go; what matters is how well you set up the fight between your hamstring and your gluteals and how deeply you challenge your glutes in the straight leg sequence.

- Don't slump your upper body by sinking into your shoulder on one side or releasing your shoulder anchor and allowing your head to droop into "vulture neck." Not only is each Fit Quickie a muscle-shaping exercise, but it's also a chance to create beautiful posture and alignment. At first it'll be challenging to remember all the details, but with a little practice, you'll get the hang of it.

- Don't swing your working leg and use momentum to accomplish the contractions, lifts, and squeezes. Make your glutes do the work!

Tips and Modifications

These tips and alternate ways to perform the exercise might help:

- You can practice Fit Quickie #4 on your elbows and knees. Simply drop from your hands to your elbows on the floor, with your elbows right beneath your shoulders and all other elements the same. This can be helpful if you have wrist issues that don't allow you to rest the weight of your upper body on your hands.

- You can also vary things by doing a portion of each set on your hands, move to your elbows, and come back to your hands again. Have fun! Mix it up!

Fit Quickie #4 is one of my favorite go-to moves if I need a quick pick-me-up or instant energizer. On the floor in front of the TV, as a quick computer break while at work in my studio, or even right before jumping into bed, I've found several easy ways to integrate this exercise into my day. And it's one of the best body shapers I know. There's a reason it's called "Gorgeous Glutes and Hamstrings."

Fit Quickie #5

TOPLESS MUFFINS

Goal/results: Target your gluteals to lift your rear end and sculpt the side of both your seat and the back of your waist; shape and strengthen the stabilizing muscles of your lower, middle, and upper back

Workout time: 5 minutes

Equipment: 12×12-inch piece of 1-inch foam padding, rolled; a 6- or 7-inch playground ball

The Problem

Doesn't the name of Fit Quickie #5—Topless Muffins—say it all? You know instantly what "muffin top" means. It's that uncomfortable roll that sits low on your waist, pushing out over the top of your jeans like a freshly baked muffin over the edges of its tin.

First, let's get one thing clear: that roll cannot be "exercised off." Reducing excess body fat stores is a result of a healthy diet combined with an active lifestyle. Yet even then—and perhaps you've experienced this—sometimes a ribbon of something remains right at the back of your waist.

The Facts

Our bodies tend to locate fat stores according to genetic predisposition and in areas where muscle is least active. The muffin top zone fulfills, for many of us, both requirements.

Even if you don't need to lose weight, you may still lack lift in this zone. You might not even have guessed that the shape of this area has anything to do with your gluteal muscles, or the muscles in your back, for that matter. But it does. And as you know, unchallenged muscles start to lose shape and lift power. That translates to lack of both on you.

What we need is something to address the unconditioned muscles that meet at this part of the body that challenges them enough to deliver lift and shape.

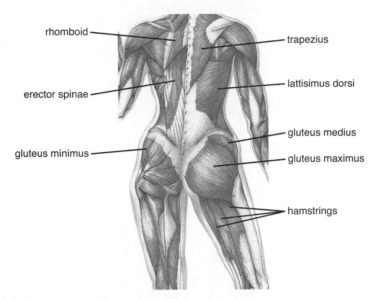

The Fit Quickie #5 advantage: lots of muscles working in concert make this little move means amazing shaping and strengthening properties for your backside.

The Fit Quickie Fix

This is one of my all-time favorite exercises. First, it targets that hard-to-reach area, the spot on the back of the waist. Combined with a low-fat diet, this exercise makes your back flow beautifully into your backside.

It also creates a lovely "dancer's curve" in the side of your hips. The muscles in this area are sorely neglected in daily activity and workouts, and by isolating and overloading the gluteus medius here, you'll have your muscles sitting up and taking notice instead of snoozing. As a bonus, you'll see a beautiful change in your hip profile.

This exercise also has a dramatic lifting-and-shaping effect on your rear end. With one or two simple tricks, you can deepen the targeting effect of this exercise quite quickly. Combined with other Fit Quickies such as #4, this is your ticket to a great backside.

How to Do It

The gluteus medius is the superstar of this exercise, with the gluteus maximus running a close second. The medius sits right on the top back outside of your hips just below your waist, right beneath the spot where fat stores seem to too easily accumulate. It's responsible for stabilizing your pelvis when you walk. It contracts to control lower-extremity movement and springs into action to steady you whenever you're thrown off balance. When the medius is weak or poorly recruited, these functions are compromised—another reason to get this muscle in good working form.

This muscle can be somewhat neglected in activities such running, cycling, and other exercises that primarily involve forward movement in a straight line—moves dominated by the quadriceps. Directly challenging your gluteus medius pays off big time in body shaping.

And it doesn't stop there. Remember, this exercise also asks you to bring the muscles low in your back at your waist gently into play, improving your posture. See why this is such a powerful combination?

 From a body-shaping standpoint, training your gluteus medius makes for some dramatic changes. Your legs can start to appear longer and start higher on your frame. As your backside tightens, saddle bags—if you have them—are reduced or can disappear altogether. And the curvy hollows that form in the sides of your hips—the "dancer's dent"—make your hips appear slimmer.

Position

Here's your starting position:

1. Sitting on the floor, place your weight on your left hip with both legs folded to your right.

2. Keeping your upper body strong, tilt your torso into your left hand, which is on the floor beside you to work with the muscles in your core and back to support your upper-body weight.

3. Fold your left leg in front of you so you have a 90-degree bend at the knee. Keep your lower leg parallel to your hips.

4. Bend your right leg at the knee so it's on the floor slightly behind your right hip. To put your right leg into position, place your hand on your right knee and gently push your right knee back until it's behind your hips.

5. With your right hand on your right hip, guide your right hip forward as you stay mindful of keeping your right knee back. Remember, you want your hips square to the front. It's this tug-of-war created between your hip forward and your knee pressed back that starts the challenge for your glutes, hamstrings, and waist. This will be present as part of your workload throughout.

6. Tighten your glutes to counter the inclination of your pelvis to roll into an all-out anterior pelvic tilt. Square your shoulders to your front lower leg on the floor in front of you. Your shoulders should form a line parallel to the one created by the knee-to-ankle of your left leg.

7. Your upper body should be completely stable, with your chest open and your abdominals engaged. As with all Fit Quickies, your upper-body position is essential with your shoulder blades anchored securely on your rib cage in back. Keep your shoulders dropped down from your ears, and use your supporting arm as a guide as you avoid letting your upper body slump into it.

8. Sandwich the rolled foam padding behind your right knee, grasping it between the top of your calf muscle and your hamstring. Flex your right foot.

9. Place the playground ball on the floor in front of your left knee, and firmly plant your right hand on the top of the ball.

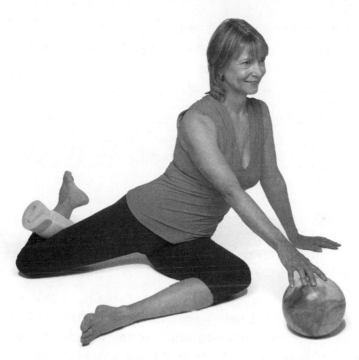

Keep your shoulders square to the leg folded in front of you, and grasp the foam pad behind your knee.

Anchors

Here are your anchor points:

- Your left hip on the floor

- The left hand on the floor to the left side of your body

- Your gripped glutes, to counter the tendency to slip into an anterior pelvic tilt

- Your abdominals, fired up to support your upper body and keep you in good form with your torso in a stable position

- The foam pad gripped behind your right knee

- Your right hand firmly pressing on the ball in front of you

- Your shoulder blades locked onto your rib cage in back

Isolate

When you're in position, you should feel as if everything is locked and loaded with muscle activation. Actually, if you feel like you have no idea how you could possibly do any movement with your right leg where it is, you're probably doing it right!

The final step is to now raise your right knee off the floor. You might find that you can barely lift your knee. The key is to keep your hips stable and your right hip locked forward while you engage your gluteals to try to pull your right knee off the floor. Yes, it's difficult, but it's not impossible.

Repetitions

Keeping your upper body stable, and without letting your back knee sneak forward even an inch, the repetitions follow a seven combinations to layer the workload and build intensity:

1. Start with 8 slow squeezes, drawing the heel of your right foot in toward your rear end. Each squeeze should take about 1 second. This is designed to fire up your hamstrings and, by virtue of your position, invite your gluteals into play right away. You'll feel it right where your gluteals and hamstrings meet at the bottom of your bottom. This is an indicator of how powerfully Fit Quickie #5 isolates and targets this area.

2. Now, keeping the foam gripped behind your right knee, slowly lift your right knee off the floor 16 times. Remember, your hips must stay forward and in position. You won't be able to raise your knee very high off the floor—maybe only $\frac{1}{2}$ inch or less.

3. Here's the squeeze-and-tease pattern for five rounds: lift, lift, lift, and hold; lift, lift, lift, and hold. Stay in your muscle and minimize the rebound, and quite quickly you'll feel the targeted area working. You should barely be moving your leg an inch up and down. Each round should take about 4 seconds.

4. Next, grasp the ball in your right hand, and extend your right arm forward while you continue with the repetitions. Adding this upper-body element increases the workload on the back of your waist—you'll feel it kick in immediately. It also deepens the work on your middle-back postural muscles as you reach forward yet keep your chest open, your shoulders down, and your shoulder blades anchored on your rib cage. Lift your right knee for 16 quick counts—still small, still in the muscle, your form still tight. Each lift should take between 1 and 2 seconds.

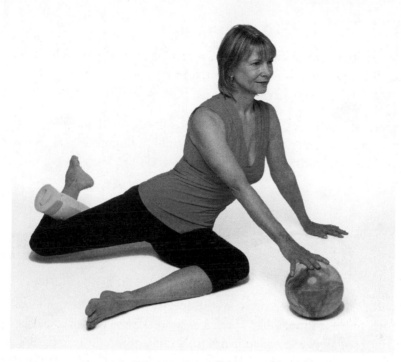

Lift your knee no more than about an inch off the floor, keeping your knee behind your hip, your hip rolled forward, and your gluteals squeezed.

 If you don't have a playground ball, you can reach your arm forward.

5. Gently pointing the toe of your right leg, use your gluteals to pull your right leg back toward the wall behind you. Keep your shoulders squared, your pelvis and hips tucked against the workload, and your right knee behind your hip and barely off the floor. Do 8 slow lifts, each about 1 second.

6. With the toes of your right foot pointing behind you, squeeze and tease with your toes to the back wall. Pull, pull, pull, and hold, for a total of 5.

7. Finish with 16 rapid repetitions of your toes reaching toward the back wall, your lower leg still wrapped close to your body as you grip the piece of foam behind your knee.

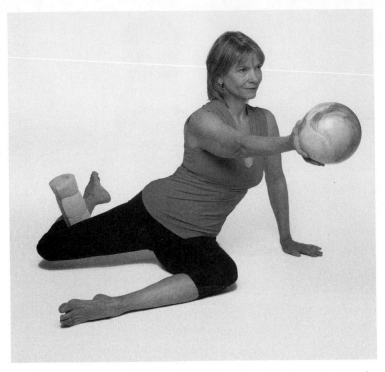

Adding an upper-body reach brings more of your upper-back muscles into play.

Then go through the entire sequence on the other side. You'll have just about 100 repetitions on each side when you're finished.

 Do as many of the repetitions in the sequences as you can while maintaining proper form. If you start to lose form or can't continue due to muscle fatigue, stop, reset yourself, and start again. It's not how many times you stop—it's how many times you jump back in that counts. You'll work your way up.

Stretch

Now for a well-deserved stretch. You'll stretch through your hip and the back of your waist on each side.

1. Sit upright and cross-legged on the floor.

2. Place your right foot on top of your left knee, putting yourself in what's called half-lotus position. Keep your ankle flexed and straight, to protect the joint. Your left foot should be under your right knee on the floor.

3. Keeping your spine long and lifted, place your fingertips on the floor beside and slightly behind you, and gently press your chest forward while extending the crown of your head to the ceiling. You'll feel this stretch immediately on the outside of your right hip; you may not even need to press forward to feel it. Breathe gently, and hold for 20 to 30 seconds.

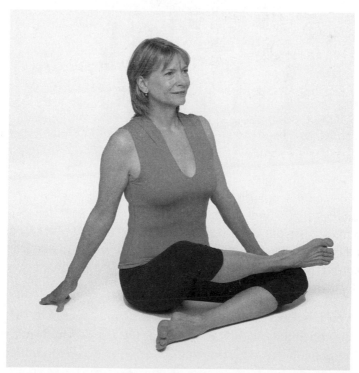

Gently press forward with your chest while reaching up with your upper body, keeping your back elongated.

If the half-lotus position is too challenging, take it down a notch by moving into a cross-legged position, dropping your top foot to the floor. As an alternative, you can sit on a bench or chair with your left foot on the floor.

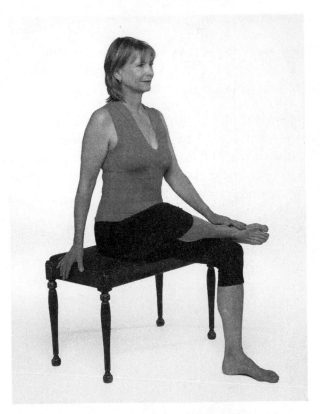

Stretching your hip while seated on a bench is an excellent alternative to doing the half-lotus stretch.

4. To stretch the back side of your waist, extend your left leg to your left and bend your right knee, bringing it in to rest the sole of your right foot high on your left inner thigh.

5. Inhale as you raise your arms overhead and lift your upper body off your hips. Rotate your upper body slightly toward your left leg, and fold your torso gently in the direction of your leg, adjusting your position as needed to target the muscles in the back side of your waist. You can extend your arms over your left leg, or let them drop to your leg and use them to gently pull your upper body into the stretch.

Either way, keep your shoulder released and down from your ear. Hold the stretch for 20 to 30 seconds.

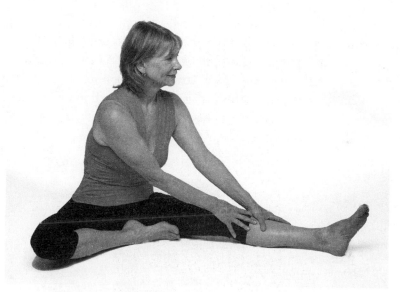

The back of your waist will also need—and enjoy—a stretch.

Repeat the entire stretch sequence for your other side.

Common Errors

Beware of these common errors while you exercise:

- Don't let the knee of your working leg sneak forward to take the exercise out of your gluteals, placing workload on your quadriceps and your hip flexor muscles on the front of your body. They always seem too willing to take over.

- Don't allow the hip of your working leg to roll backward, again an effort by your quadriceps and hip flexors to do the work.

- Don't collapse your upper body from the beautiful and elegant lift you started with to help you muscle through the job. Repeatedly cycle your attention through your posture and form, and line up everything again, if you need to.

Tips and Modifications

These tips and alternate ways to perform the exercise might help:

- If you find it impossible at first to even budge the knee of your working leg off the floor, you can adjust your position. Lean your upper body farther to the side opposite your working leg by moving your hand farther away from your body—be careful to keep your spine lifted and as straight as possible. You can even drop to your elbow on the side, onto either a yoga block or the floor. Know that this changes the working angle of the exercise somewhat, and you want to progress to being on your hand unless you can't because of back or hip issues.

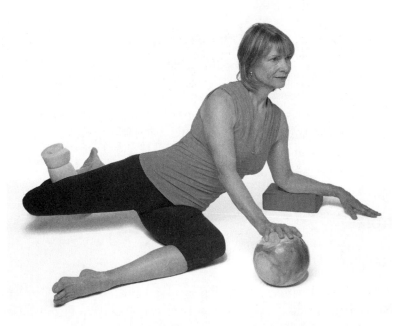

To help you work your way up to this exercise, you can lower your upper body and use the support of a yoga block.

- Unless you're already familiar with other variations of this exercise, you might not be able to complete all the repetitions at first. That's fine! Do as many repetitions as you can, with each variation in correct form. If you find yourself slipping out of form—which happens when the muscles are too challenged to continue and they try to sneak your body out of correct working position—stop, realign your body, and jump back in again. Each time you do this exercise, you'll be able to do a few more repetitions. Just work your way up.

- If grasping the foam padding *and* doing the lifts on your working leg is too difficult at first, eliminate the foam pad while you get the hang of the movement. (Actually, this is another variation and delivers results.) Having the foam pad in place adds the extra challenge of your hamstring backed up to your gluteals in contraction, and that's one thing that sets Fit Quickie #5 apart from similar exercises. Just add the foam pad later when you get the hang of the exercise.

- You can stretch each side before moving on to the other. The stretch feels so good that you might not want to wait until the end!

If ever there was one standout, super-sculpting move, it just might be Fit Quickie #5. Believe it or not, it's also super-relaxing. There's something about the position, the elegantly controlled tiny moves, and the stretch at the end. Sometimes I do it right before bed so I can climb under the covers with that all-worked-out-and-stretched feeling. Hands down, it's the most powerful upper-seat and back-of-waist shaper I've found, and it provides a powerful lift to your entire posterior as well. When you combine it with a healthy, slimming, and satisfying diet, I guarantee you'll be pleased with the results.

Fit Quickie #6
THIG WARRIORS

Goal/results: Shape and strengthen your quadriceps; stabilize your knees; improve your balance, coordination, and posture

Workout time: Less than 4 minutes

Equipment: High-back chair, dance bar, or countertop edge; 6- or 7-inch playground ball

The Problem

Unshaped, soft thighs and weak knee joints present a multitude of postural, functional strength, and aesthetic problems. Your inner quadriceps muscles are often weaker than your outer quadriceps muscles. Other imbalances prevail as well.

If you want to sculpt beautiful legs, have rock-solid thighs, create better balance in your quadriceps, and stabilize your knees, Fit Quickie #6 is a powerful addition to your workout plan.

The Facts

The quadriceps femoris is a group of four muscles: the vastus lateralis, vastus intermedius, vastus medialis, and rectus femoris.

The "quads," as they're called, have a sweeping expanse, extending all the way down through your knee. One of them, the rectus femoris, crosses both your knee and your hip joint. It's the largest muscle group in your body, which means that every time you challenge your quads with exercise—as you do here—you also ramp up calorie burn.

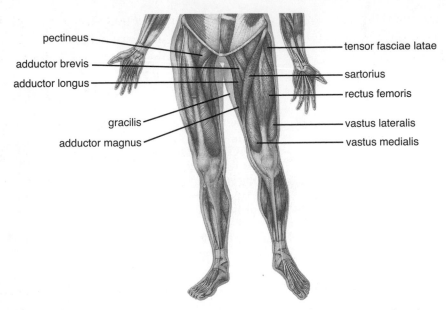

pectineus

adductor brevis

adductor longus

gracilis

adductor magnus

tensor fasciae latae

sartorius

rectus femoris

vastus lateralis

vastus medialis

The quadriceps group includes four muscles and is surrounded by several supporting players.

All four quadriceps are powerful extensors of your knee and play a crucial role in walking, running, jumping, and squatting. Because the rectus femoris is attached to the ilium, the uppermost and largest bone in your pelvis, it also flexes your hip. The quadriceps muscles also stabilize your knee joints when you're moving about.

With all these responsibilities, you can see why it's crucial to keep your quadriceps team in good working form—for function as well as beauty.

 If this exercise connects with your inner dancer, it's with good reason. The moves are inspired by my dance class patterns for building strong, shapely, long-striding thighs.

The Fit Quickie Fix

The Thigh Warriors sequence targets your quadriceps muscle group. By conditioning and shaping your quads, you not only create an aesthetic flow from the front of your hip all the way down to your knee, but you also build healthier knee joints and infuse more vitality into all your movements involving your lower body.

The intense, nonimpact contractions of this exercise very effectively create strength and balance in your quadriceps. Although your inner quads usually lag behind your outer quads in strength, Position 1 of Fit Quickie #6 addresses this imbalance specifically with the use of the ball pressed between your thighs.

 The controlled movement of this exercise builds knee stability safely by strengthening the muscles around the knee joint. This is enhanced when you raise to your heels during this move. This lifting off your heels and rising onto the balls of your feet further engages your calf muscles, which, in turn, assist in knee stabilization. It's a win-win-win.

How to Do It

You do Thigh Warriors in two positions: first with your feet parallel and then with your feet turned out in what is called second position. Don't worry if you're not familiar with "second position." I explain exactly how to do it.

Position 1

Here's your starting position:

1. Stand facing your support, with your feet parallel and directly below your hips, 4 or 5 inches apart.

2. Now get your upper body lined up. Lift the weight of your ribs off your hips, lengthen your spine, open your chest, and have your shoulders back and anchored on your shoulder blades. Your abdominals should be firm as you create your anchored neutral position.

3. Place the playground ball between your legs at mid-thigh. The ball should be slightly deflated so you can get a good grip on it.

4. Completely straighten your legs and come up high on the balls of your feet, keeping your ankle joints straight.

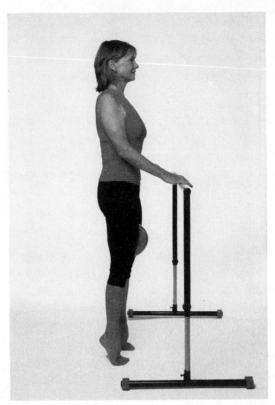

Create a strong start by getting your body properly lined up before the workload.

5. In a controlled fashion, keeping a firm grip on the ball and staying perfectly aligned with your posture vertical from your hips to your shoulders, drift down by bending your knees while staying high on your toes.

6. Let your knees drift forward directly over your second toe. You'll feel your quadriceps coming into play right away. Maintaining good upper-body form, lower your only as far as you can without compromising your upper-body position and knee joints. Go to your "personal challenge point," or the place where you're aware that your muscles are going to be in for some interesting work and your knees are still up to the job. Only go as deep as possible while paying attention to your specific joint needs. This position is very stabilizing to the knee joint, but if you feel sensitivity in your knees, come back up slightly, decreasing the amount of bend in your knees.

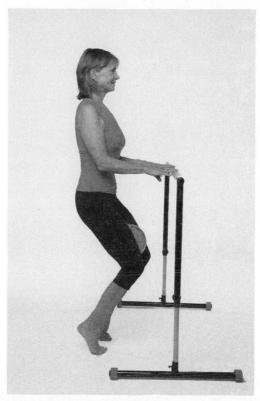

In position 1, lower to your point of challenge. Be sure to move within a range of motion that allows for success, not to the point that you can't maintain your posture or experience pain or discomfort.

 Don't be surprised if your legs start to shake a little when you drop into work position. This means your muscles are already being challenged, and that's a good thing. Go for the quiver!

7. Recheck that your upper body is lined up correctly, and reset as needed before going on. You should still have your shoulders right below your ears, your gaze forward and level, your shoulders stacked directly over your hips, and your pelvis in anchored position. The tendency will be to release your glutes, allowing your tailbone to lift in back, placing your pelvis in an excessive anterior tilt. You'll need to grip your glutes slightly and engage your abdominals to maintain correct alignment. Check in a mirror to be sure you're not allowing your tailbone to lift in back. Soon you'll you get the feel of the position. Stay high on the balls of your feet because you're ready to begin the repetitions.

Anchors

Here are your anchor points:

- The balls of your feet on the floor

- Your hand lightly on the chair or bar to stabilize

- Your thighs locked on the ball

- Your shoulder blades anchored on your back

- Your anchored pelvis, with your abdominals and gluteals engaged

Isolate

You've achieved isolation of the quadriceps by lowering into position. Your work is already underway!

Repetitions

Here's how Fit Quickie #6 works:

1. In the lowest position you can go while maintaining correct posture and with respect to knee safety and comfort, hold for a count of 8 seconds. During this time, recheck the position of your upper body and continue to press lower into the position as your strength and knees allow.

2. Keeping a gentle grip on the ball and still staying high on your toes, slowly drop down an inch, and then another inch, and come right back up as little as possible: down, down, up, and hold. Your goal is to stay low in your challenge zone and then drop lower for a couple counts before coming back to that low position again. Don't return to a full stand unless you absolutely need a break. Do this pattern for 8 rounds; each round should take about 4 seconds.

3. Now, moving up the tempo, do very small movements down, up, down, up, keeping as low as you can in good shoulder-to-hip position and using a small range of motion. Do 20 repetitions, with each rep taking about 1 second.

4. Rise and move into position 2 for the next set of repetitions.

Position 2

At this point, you're done with the ball. In this next series of repetitions, you change the position of your feet, and the workload on your thighs shifts a little, too. You'll feel it in your outer quadriceps.

Here's your starting position:

1. Place your feet flat on the floor in second position, or with your heels touching and your toes pointing out at a diagonal. You'll create a 90-degree angle with your feet, extending from your heels.

2. Reconnect with your posture, straighten your legs, and come up high on your toes again. From here, walk your feet in together so that your heels are touching. Again, slowly lower into your challenge zone, letting your knees drift out directly over the midline of your foot and your toes in their outturned position. Keep your heels pressed together. Be sure you're not letting your knees roll in; keep them pointing straight over your toes.

3. Check that your upper body is lined up correctly, and reset yourself if necessary before continuing. You should still have your shoulders below your ears, your gaze forward and level, your shoulders stacked directly over your hips, and your spine neutral, with all its natural curves in place.

As you lower into your challenge zone, your body might want to release your glutes, allowing your tailbone to lift in back and placing your pelvis in an excessive anterior tilt. You'll need to grip your glutes slightly and engage your abdominals to maintain correct alignment. Until you get a feel for the position, check in a mirror to be sure you aren't allowing your tailbone to lift in back. If necessary, decrease the bend in your knees to restore proper form—always a priority!

Repeat the repetitions you did for position 1 in this new, out-turned position.

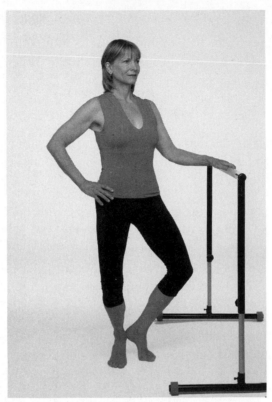

In position 2, keep your heels pressed tightly together while you lower to your point of challenge with your knees correctly aligned.

You can always restart and do another set of each of these, if you like. Be sure to watch for and avoid letting your shoulders sneak forward to allow you to lean on the support. Also, don't let them fall backward to save you from the workload. Keep your ribs, hips, and shoulders aligned. Keep your abdominals engaged. Imagining a slight forward fold at your waist without shifting your shoulders forward may be helpful.

Stretch

Now for the stretch:

1. Stand with your left foot on the floor, your knee slightly bent.

2. Raise your right foot off the floor and bend your right knee, pointing the toes of your right foot behind you.

3. Reach back with your right hand, and grasp the heel, ankle, or even pant leg of your right foot—whatever you can reach. You'll feel the stretch right away through your quadriceps. Avoid pulling your right heel in hard. Instead, think of moving your right foot toward the wall behind you as you facilitate the stretch with your right hand. Keep your right knee pointing down to the floor, and don't let it drift out to the side. While holding the stretch, keep your pelvis tucked under to extend the stretch all the way up the top of your thigh and into the front of your hip joint. Keep your standing leg softly bent. Hold the stretch for 20 to 30 seconds.

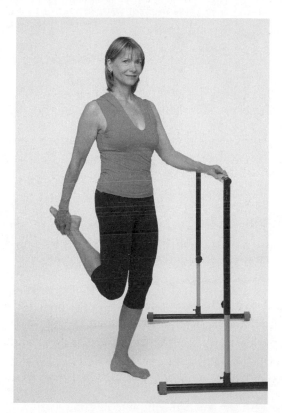

During the stretch, keep the knee of your bent leg close to your standing leg.

Doesn't that feel good? Now repeat it on the other side.

Common Errors

Beware of these common errors while you exercise:

- Don't release your upper-body alignment to compensate for the balance challenge of correct position as you lower into your challenge zone.

- Don't allow for too much range of motion in steps 2 and 3 of the repetitions. These are measured in inches and shouldn't be anything close to a squat-type motion. No deeply bent knees—that's too stressful on your knee joints. Stay focused in your challenge zone, and work your quadriceps safely.

- Don't grasp and lean into your support. It's there as a structural alignment tool, so only a light touch, please!

- Don't drop your heels too close to the floor. Stay high on the balls of your feet.

- Don't bend your knees to the point of pain. If you have persistent knee issues, don't allow your knees to drift beyond the ends of your toes, or avoid the exercise.

Tips and Modifications

These tips and alternate ways to perform the exercise might help:

- If position 1 provides too much challenge for your knees, do all the repetitions in position 2, or vice versa. This exercise stabilizes the knee joint, and my clients and students who have knee issues have benefitted from this exercise. At the same time, it's imperative that you be respectful of your own anatomical concerns.

- Don't be afraid of the shake in the thigh muscles when you get underway.

- Start with the repetitions you can complete in good form, and then work your way up. There's plenty of room for progression here as you vary the number of repetitions and the depth you drop into working position.

- If you need some padding under the balls of your feet, stand on a foam pad or carpet.

- Be sure to stand true on the balls of your feet with a straight ankle joint. Check that you're not letting your ankle roll outward or inward.

- When reaching to grasp your foot behind you to stretch your thigh, feel free to use a strap if your ankle seems too far away to grasp. Simply loop a belt or length of webbing over your ankle to gently move into the stretch.

See why I call these Thigh Warriors?

Fit Quickie #7
KICKSTAND CORE CHALLENGE

Goal/results: Isolate and strengthen your abdominal muscles to help shape your waist, challenge your core musculature, and improve your posture

Workout time: Less than 3 minutes

Equipment: Two 6- or 7-inch playground balls, slightly deflated

The Problem

As discussed in Fit Quickie #1, when it comes to your abdominal profile, there are two players: unconditioned muscles and excess body fat. You need to challenge your abdominal muscles to shape and strengthen them, and to restore their girdling power. But your hard work won't show unless and until you also reduce your body fat stores. For that, you need to look at what you eat. (More on that later.)

The Facts

The good news is that you don't need lots of specific abdominal work. The face of abdominal training as we know it is changing. According to Stuart McGill, PhD, spine biomechanics specialist, the core musculature—of which your abdominals are a part, along with your gluteals and several muscles in your back—functions differently from those of your limbs. Your core muscles are not only movers, they also co-contract and serve as stabilizers in a synergistic fashion. As you train your abdominal muscles, you need to take this into consideration.

If your current workout routine has you doing extraordinarily high repetitions of crunches, sit-ups, or half-hour "ab" routines, that's about to change. It isn't necessary, nor is it desirable. It's far better to select a few specific, powerful strategies and pay more attention to core-challenging exercises, cardiovascular activity, and dietary plan. Even 10 minutes on a stationary bike does more to trim your waist than the same amount of time devoted to traditional sit-ups. Doing an overabundance of abdominal exercise is probably a carry-over of spot-reduction thinking, and it's high time we change that line of thought. Remember, there's no such thing as spot-specific fat reduction. Fat stored in your subcutaneous tissue, beneath your skin, belongs to your entire body. Just as fuel in the gas tank powers your entire car, your body fat storage provides energy for your entire body.

Perhaps the most compelling evidence refuting the myth of spot reduction comes from a study conducted by Katch and team at the University of Massachusetts in 1984. In this study, subjects participated in a vigorous abdominal exercise training program for 4 weeks. Each participant performed a total of 5,000 sit-ups over the course of the research project. Fat biopsies were taken from the subjects' abdomens, upper backs, and buttocks both before and after the exercise program.

The results of the study revealed that their fat stores did decrease, but fat reduction was similar in all three sites, not just in the abdominal region. This may help explain why spot reducing sometimes appears to work. If you expend enough calories, you'll lose fat from your entire body—your storage tank. This includes any specifically targeted area.

 Although fat is lost or gained throughout your entire body, according to your genetics, apparently the last areas to become lean are those areas where an individual tends to gain fat first. In other words, last hired, first fired. As for gender differences, generally men find the abdomen area the most challenging to reduce fat, while for women, the hips, buttocks, thighs, and upper arms present the greatest fat-loss challenge. These are general observations, as there are variations among individual people.

The Fit Quickie Fix

Along with Fit Quickie #1, Kickstand Core Challenge is about the only type of specific ab exercise I do. The rest I leave to the abdominal-targeting effects of push-ups, planks, and other core-stabilizing exercises that require balance. (More about this in Fit Quickie #11.)

Another research-driven Fit Quickie, this exercise zooms right in on your abdominals quite quickly when you're in correct position. The American Council on Exercise conducted a study to examine 13 of the most common exercises for the abdominal muscles. Using electromyography (EMG), they ranked exercises based on the amount of EMG activity recorded in the abdominal area.

The results? Overwhelmingly, the exercises that generated the most abdominal muscle activity were those that required constant abdominal stabilization, and abdominal crunches on a stability ball ranked the best overall. Add some body rotation to target your obliques, those waist-cinching muscles that wrap around the sides of your middle, and you've got targeted body shaping at its best.

The benefits gained by using a stability ball and the important trunk rotation are carried forward into Kickstand Core Challenge, with three important improvements in safety and effectiveness. First, the smaller playground ball you use better conforms to the natural lumbar curve in your back than a large ball, delivering better lumbar support and safety. Also, this exercise places your torso in a supported yet slightly destabilized position, bringing all the muscles of your abdomen into play right from the start. Perfect. Finally, repeated deep flexing of the lumbar spine is removed from the equation, protecting the discs of your lower back by implementing an isometric hold with your back held in neutral spine position.

Training your abdominals, you might have noticed, is a different experience from training other muscles in your body. It can take you longer to connect with the "feel" of training these muscles than with any others. The main reason for this slower response is that your abdominal muscles always work together. Your transversus abdominis muscle, deep below your belt line; your obliques that wrap around the sides of your torso for stability, flexion, and rotation; and your more superficial rectus abdominis, your "six-pack" muscle, all work as a team rather than act alone. So it might take a little more time to send the signal from your brain to your muscles for targeted exercise, especially when those muscles are weak. And with Fit Quickie #7, as with all core-stabilizing abdominal exercises, expect a more comprehensive challenge to your abdominal area rather than a small targeted burn.

With the way I've designed this exercise to isolate and overload those muscles, combined with a little practice, you'll be able to zero in on your abdominals and feel them just seconds into the work. For effective abdominal training, I emphasize body position and movement proficiency. You can yield the best results by focusing on your technique and the proper positioning of your body.

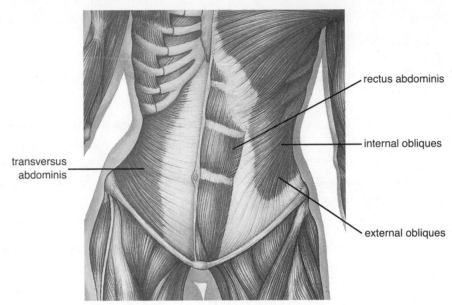

rectus abdominis

internal obliques

transversus
abdominis

external obliques

Fit Quickie #7 brings all your abdominal muscles into play while recruiting many other core muscles as well.

Do these exercises with *control*. Make each second count.

How to Do It

There's growing concern that traditional abdominal workouts such as sit-ups and crunches, which have you repeatedly performing deep curls forward at the waist, flattening your back, place potentially damaging stress on the discs of your lumbar spine. Remember, the spine has a natural curve in the lumbar region, and extended and repeated movement against that curve can be counterproductive.

The position of this exercise changes that. The support of the ball at your lower back keeps your spine in its natural curve to challenge your abdominals, and core, in a way that's safe for your back. Eliminating the deep flexion that comes with traditional sit-ups enables you to stay focused on maintaining optimal spine position while your body scrambles to recruit your abdominals and other core muscles to keep you stabilized. You'll feel this challenge through your abdominal muscles quite quickly.

Position 1

Here's your starting position:

1. Sit on the floor with your knees bent and your feet flat on the floor in front of you, hip width apart.

2. Grasp one ball between your knees. This gives you another point of anchor and helps you maintain correct position. It also helps stabilize your lower body and brings your inner thighs gently into play. Be mindful of keeping your upper body strong, your chest open, and your shoulders in proper alignment and wrapped around your rib cage in back throughout the exercise.

Full-range sit-ups and crunches work your hip flexors more than they work your abdominals. You want to keep the challenge in your abdominals as much as possible.

3. Place the other ball behind you at the back of your waist, where it will take the shape of the natural curve of your lower back— essentially, it'll serve as your kickstand, hence the name of the exercise.

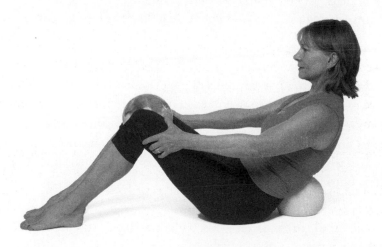

Position one ball at the back of your waist for excellent lumbar support and another between your knees as an anchor.

Anchors

Here are your anchor points:

- Your feet on the floor

- Your thighs with a firm grasp on the ball

- Your lower back's contact with the ball

- Your shoulders pressed down from your ears and your shoulder blades anchored on your rib cage in back

Isolate

While keeping contact with the ball at the back of your waist for lumbar support, and using your hands at your knees as guide, lower your body gently to the ball. Remember, the ball should be partially deflated to allow for stable positioning. You should feel as if you're leaning slightly into the ball for support, but you're still required to recruit your abdominal muscles to hold yourself in position. Your abdominal muscles will immediately scramble into play, fulfilling their function as stabilizers. This is exactly what you want.

Engage your abdominals just enough so you aren't lying over the ball with your body weight, but maintaining correct alignment of your spine, including the lumbar curve.

Repetitions

Here's what to do:

1. In the isolate position you just achieved, without any other movement, continue to breathe at a normal cadence while turning your attention toward maintaining your position with isometric contraction through your abdominals. Hold for a count of 10 to 30 seconds.

If you can't make it for 30 seconds, hold only as long as you're able to maintain correct position through your upper body and not collapse all your weight into the ball. If you start to lose proper form after just a few seconds, release your position by pulling yourself with your arms on your legs to bring your body to sitting position.

Position 2

Next, you're going to move to a second, rotation position to more specifically target your obliques:

1. From position 1, let yourself now lean your weight into the ball at your back while keeping proper spine alignment as you move into position 2. Lift your rib cage from your hips gently to create slightly more space in your midsection, and anchor your left elbow on the floor directly beneath your left shoulder as a second kickstand of support. Reach with your right hand to the outside of your left thigh just this side of your knee, or to wherever you can reach on your outer left thigh, while extending your left leg straight. Keep your anchor point against the ball at your back and knees. You're simply opening the angle of your knee joint by straightening your leg on the left side. This involves your hip flexor muscles to some extent, yet you'll also notice this extension adds an extra load to your work at the side of your waist.

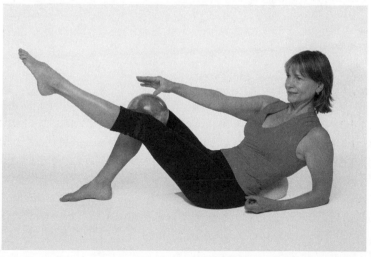

When rotating your torso into position 2, you'll feel the addition of the workload in the side of your waist.

2. With your right arm, gently pull your weight away from the ball. Simultaneously press your left elbow into the floor to assist in lifting your weight slightly away from the ball at your back so you're no longer leaning on it yet you're still utilizing it for lumbar support as in position 1. Keep your upper body strong, your chest open, and your shoulders in proper alignment and wrapped around your rib cage in back throughout the exercise.

3. In the isolate position you just achieved, without any other movement, continue to breathe at a normal cadence while turning your attention toward maintaining your position with isometric contraction through your abdominals. If you can maintain proper integrity of your spinal position, you can release your right hand from your left leg and reach forward past your left knee. If the extended leg gives you too much workload, start with both feet on the floor and work your way up. Hold for a count of 10 to 30 seconds.

Hold only as long as you're able to maintain correct position through your upper body and not collapse all your weight onto the ball. Should you start to lose proper form after just a few seconds, release your position.

Repeat on the other side. And feel free to repeat all three positions for another round.

Stretch

Now for your stretch:

1. Release both balls, and roll onto your stomach, with your legs extended behind you.

2. Place your elbows on the floor beneath or slightly in front of your shoulders, yet close in by your side.

3. Allow your abdominals to release, open, and stretch. This also stretches the front of your spine.

Fit Quickie #7 is one of those exercises that works faster as you get better at it. It's a body profile changer. And watch how it affects your posture and energy, too.

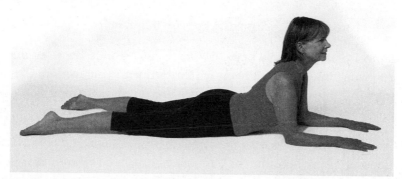

Move gently and carefully into the stretch. Keep your feet on the floor and your legs relaxed.

Common Errors

Beware of these common errors while you exercise:

- Don't bounce your back against the ball in the style of abdominal crunches. There's no release or stretch of your abdominals during the sequence. You've placed them in a working position, keeping you stabilized while your back rests against the ball.

- Don't allow your shoulders to collapse forward, releasing them from their anchor on your rib cage in back and shifting the workload to your arms and shoulders. Maintain form throughout—and if you can't continue with the correct form, stop, regain your position, and pick up the count again.

- Don't sink into the shoulder of your working side during position 2. Stay strong in your upper body—and if you do lose form, stop, reconnect, and jump in again.

- Don't allow your head to jut forward to help with the work. Keep your neck long. If you feel excess tension or fatigue in your neck, stop, turn your head from side to side to release, and then resume.

Tips and Modifications

These tips and alternate ways to perform the exercise might help:

- In position 1, if you can hold in good form for 30 seconds, try releasing your hold from your thighs and simply reach forward with your arms in the direction of your knees. However, be sure you haven't resorted to creating a curl position, compromising the neutral position in your lower back.

- Don't lean your torso back over the top of the ball. You should come back no farther than anchored neutral position of your spine. Also avoid extending your lower back by lying over the ball. If you start to bend back too far as you tire, stop. Gradually increase your time in hold position only as your strength allows while maintaining correct spinal position.

- If the torso rotation sections where your leg is extended present too much of a challenge for your abdominals to keep correct form, keep both feet on the floor to begin with and work your way up.

- If you don't have two balls, you can switch out the one placed between your knees for a pillow.

Practice this exercise three or four times a week. At first, you might find that you can only hold the correct position for a few seconds. Actually, that's a good thing because it probably means you're in correct position, placing the challenge on your core. Challenge intensity trumps time in position every time.

Fit Quickie #8
TUSH TIGHTENERS

Goal/results: Isolate and strengthen your gluteal muscles to reshape your rear end and improve your posture; improve your hamstring flexibility

Workout time: $4\frac{1}{2}$ minutes

Equipment: One 6- or 7-inch playground ball; webbing, belt, or strap for the stretch; 5- to 15-pound dumbbells

The Problem

How ironic that the largest muscle in your body spends most of the day literally doing nothing as you sit. Most people's gluteals are underdeveloped because of how much of the day they spend in a seated position. Combined with lack of deep challenge to these big muscles—which are all over your backside—it's no wonder we've lost shape, strength, and stability back there. And as you know, weak gluteal muscles also contribute to belly pooch and back pain.

In addition, your hamstrings on the backs of your thighs tend to be tight, and most people need to develop hamstring flexibility. For this reason, I've added my favorite hamstring-gluteal stretch to this chapter to piggyback this exercise.

The Facts

The gluteals, as you know from Fit Quickie #4, are a group of three muscles—the gluteus maximus, gluteus medius, and gluteus minimus—located at the back of your hips. The gluteus maximus is the largest and most superficial muscle of the group; along with fat stores, it contributes most of the mass of your buttocks.

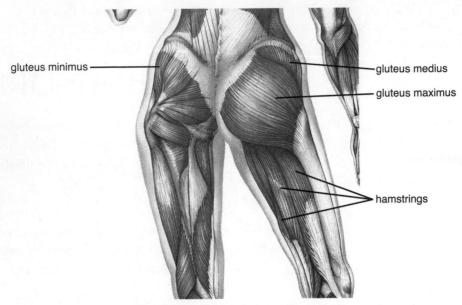

gluteus minimus

gluteus medius

gluteus maximus

hamstrings

The gluteals are one of the largest yet laziest muscle groups. The good news is,
the gluteals respond quickly to a resistance challenge.

Your glutes are responsible for hip extension, such as when you extend your leg behind you
as you stride, and lateral rotation, such as any time you rotate your leg or hip away from the
center of your body. They also assist in keeping your body in an upright position.

The Fit Quickie Fix

Fit Quickie #8 is a quick-and-easy way to get your gluteals firing because it isolates and
targets them quite quickly. Believe me, you'll see within seconds where this exercise got its
name.

This exercise is a variation of yoga's bridge position, with some distinct differences. Instead
of raising your hips way off the floor as in a yoga bridge, you keep your rib cage dropped
close to the floor during the gluteal contractions. Your upper body stays relaxed yet anchored
while you focus the workload through your rear end. This keeps your back out of the work
and puts all the workload in your gluteal muscles, which is right where you want it. You'll lift
your rear end only a few inches off the floor.

This basic position is a powerful way to isolate and strengthen your gluteals. By doing this exercise correctly, you'll also find that it's a good core-stability and -strengthening exercise that subtly targets your abdominal muscles. The position is also considered a basic rehabilitative exercise for improving core and spinal stabilization.

I like to use this exercise in three ways. I often use it to finish a workout. This move is fun, and I always look forward to it after the rest of my hard work. It's actually great motivation and incentive. And when done correctly, it relieves tension in the lower back, so although it provides a muscle challenge, it also has a relaxing effect.

If you don't want to leave it to the end of a workout, this exercise is also an effective way to tire your gluteal muscles so that any other work you do there afterward really works deeper into the muscle. For example, completing Fit Quickie #8 before Fit Quickie #4 makes you very aware, from the first downbeat of Fit Quickie #4, what muscles you're targeting.

In addition, this exercise is an instant invigorator. The next time you're feeling sluggish and need a boost, get on the floor and do this exercise. No warm-up required. In less than 5 minutes, you'll burn some extra calories, get charged up and energized to tackle your projects, and feel an instant spring in your step. It works every time.

How to Do It

You're going to need your playground ball and a belt or strap for the finishing stretch. If you've worked your way up to the addition of extra resistance, have those dumbbells handy, too. We're going to use 2 positions, with 6 sequences in each position.

Position 1

Here's your starting position:

1. Lie on your back on the floor, with your knees bent and your feet flat on the floor a comfortable distance from your hips. Your feet should be about hip width apart, with your toes straight ahead.

2. Place the ball between your thighs, and grasp it firmly. Lengthen your spine and relax your back on the floor, with your arms by your sides or folded across your rib cage. Relax your upper body while you focus the workload through your glutes. Remember to keep your rib cage dropped to the floor during the gluteal contractions.

3. Connect with your posture and alignment as you do while in standing Fit Quickies: your shoulders are relaxed down and away from your ears, your spine and neck are lengthened, and your are shoulders back—don't let them sneak forward to help with the work.

4. If you're using extra weight, place the dumbbells across the front of your pelvis. This provides you with extra resistance. Start with no weight. You can then begin using a low weight and work your way up from there. Hold the weights in place with your hands, keeping your arms as relaxed as possible.

Anchors

Here are your anchor points:

- Your feet on the floor

- The ball gripped between your thighs

- Your back all the way to the bottom of your rib cage and up through the top of your head on the floor

- Your shoulder blades locked on your rib cage in back, your shoulders pressed down from your ears

Isolate

To isolate your gluteals, drive your heels into the floor and squeeze your gluteals to raise your rear end off the floor just a couple inches, keeping your rib cage down.

The grip in your glutes is your isolation. Although your hamstrings will be fired up, by keeping your rib cage low—along with placing the focus of your attention through the gluteal contraction—you're able to keep them released as much as possible. Stay mindful while lifting your hips off the floor to initiate the work from your gluteals.

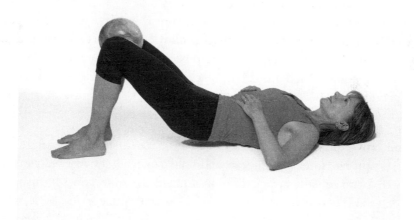

Keep your rib cage dropped to the floor as you tighten your gluteals to lift them a couple inches off the floor.

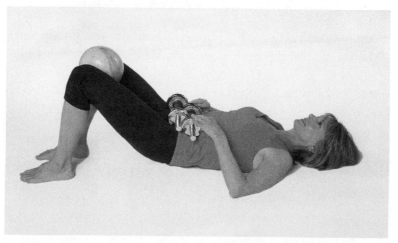

When you're ready to add more resistance to this exercise, start with a light weight and add more as you progress.

Repetitions

Here's how Fit Quickie # 8 works:

1. Start with small squeezes with a tiny range of motion. Your hips barely move while you stay close the top of your raised hip position. Your hips won't touch the floor during this step. Squeeze and release for 20 repetitions. Each contraction takes about 1 second.

2. Utilizing a slightly wider range of motion, allow your hips to move to the floor between squeezes. Be careful, however, to keep your rib cage down. Your hips won't come up any higher than before, but they'll drop lower during each rep. This will feel really good to your back, and because it's following the tiny initial squeezes, you'll feel this moving more deeply into your muscles. Do 20 repetitions, each about 1 second.

3. Now for one of my favorites, the squeeze and tease. Using a tiny range of motion as in step 1, squeeze, squeeze, squeeze, and hold; squeeze, squeeze, squeeze, and hold. Notice that you actually have a lot more time in the squeeze with this move than in the release. That's how it should be. Do 5 sets of squeeze and tease, with each squeeze taking about 1 second and each squeeze and hold taking 2 seconds.

4. Next you'll do rapid isometric squeezes at the top of the step 1 position. Check that your rib cage is still down, your upper body is dropped into the floor, and your face is relaxed. Do 20 repetitions, about 2 per second.

5. Finally, complete an isometric hold in step 1 position without any release for 10 counts. You should feel this deep in your gluteals. Don't let those eager hamstrings hijack the job!

Position 2

Move into position 2 before continuing:

1. Let your hips drop to the floor, and release the ball while you reposition your feet for position 2.

2. Move your feet apart from each other to a wide stance, about 2 to 2½ feet apart. This places the workload more to the outside of your gluteals. You'll still be targeting your gluteus maximus, but you'll also be moving more into your gluteus medius.

3. Reconnect with your upper-body alignment and anchors. Drive your heels into the floor so that your rear end is again an inch or two off the floor, your rib cage is down, and your arms are relaxed, your shoulders anchored and your neck long.

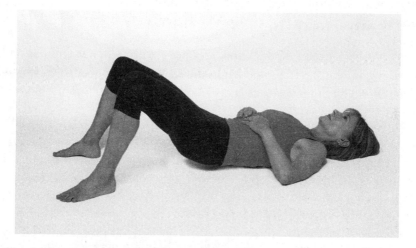

In position 2, place your feet about 2½ feet apart, shifting the emphasis to your gluteus maximus and your gluteus medius.

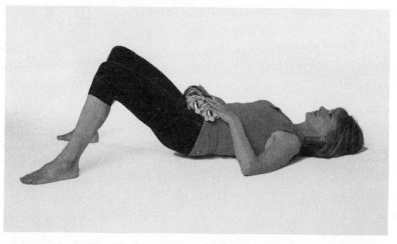

If you're adding extra resistance with weights, put them in place across your hips before you lift your pelvis off the floor.

Repeat the repetition steps 1 through 5 in this new position. By the time you're done with both positions, you'll know exactly where your gluteals are.

Stretch

Now for a well-deserved stretch:

1. Lie on your back on the floor, with your knees bent and your feet flat on the floor just below your hips. Before you begin the stretch, reconnect with your upper-body alignment and let your head, shoulders, and rib cage drop into the floor.

2. Use a belt or strap for this stretch, which helps deepen the hamstring and gluteal stretch. With your right foot on the floor and your right knee bent, loop the belt around the arch of your left foot. Nudge your right foot a little farther away from your body, and extend your left leg straight. At this point, the important thing is to straighten your left leg—you haven't even started to the stretch, so it shouldn't be extending toward the ceiling just yet.

3. When your leg is straight, exhale as you gently invite your left leg in toward your chest. Bring in your leg only as far as you can without bending your knee. Otherwise, you take the stretch out of your hamstrings, which is where you want to focus. Keep your palms facing each other and your shoulders down from your ears as you let your arms open to your sides, creating a big circle with your arms to invite your leg in so your shoulders don't tighten. During the entire stretch, keep your upper body anchored on the floor. Avoid leveraging into position by pressing your right foot into the floor, which tends to abort the stretch somewhat. It doesn't matter how high you bring that leg; what matters is keeping your leg straightened, the rest of your body in good anchored alignment, and feeling the stretch. Hold the stretch, breathing gently, for 20 to 30 seconds.

Now repeat the stretch on your right leg.

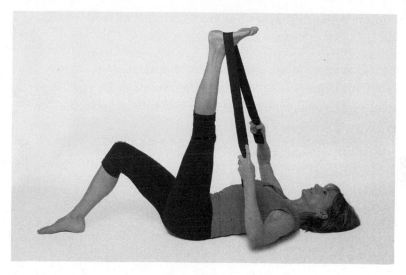

Be sure to straighten your leg before you even think about challenging it with a stretch.

Common Errors

Beware of these common errors while you exercise:

- Don't allow for too much range of motion in the gluteal contractions. Remember, in several steps, these squeezes are tiny and sharp. When instructions are for "full range," you're still moving only a few inches.

- Don't allow your shoulders to press forward toward the ceiling, releasing them from their anchor on the floor as if to help with the job. Maintain your form throughout; if you find it impossible to continue with correct form, stop, regain your position, and pick up the repetitions again.

- Don't lift the bottom of your rib cage off the floor. This can cause lower-back tension. Keep your rib cage dropped down so you can isolate the work into your lower body.

- Don't move too much of the work into your hamstrings. They need to be slightly engaged, but you want to be aware of releasing them as much as possible.

- Don't tighten through your jaw and face. Let them relax!

- During the stretch, don't pull on the stretching leg strap with hunched shoulders and lots of arm power. Rather, keep your arms in an open arc with your back anchored. This helps you avoid creating tension through your upper body, inhibiting your overall focus on flexibility and relaxation with the stretch.

Tips and Modifications

These tips and alternate ways to perform the exercise might help:

- If you want to make this more of a hamstring exercise, simply nudge your feet farther away from your hips, in either position, and you'll instantly feel the workload move down your legs. However, you won't be able to rise as high off the floor this way as in the original positions.

- If the weights on your hips seem like too much, you can leave them out and still get an excellent gluteal challenge. Always be sure you have the technique down before you add extra resistance. After a few practice sessions, you can start with a light weight of 3 to 5 pounds and work your way up from there.

- To increase the challenge even more, as an advanced alternative, you can lift one foot off the floor and extend your leg toward the ceiling. Be sure, however, to keep your hips square and not let the hip of your extended leg dip toward the ground, compromising your back. If you're doing the extended leg variation, don't use any weights on the front of your hips.

Isn't Fit Quickie #8 great? Don't you feel reenergized and zippy?

Fit Quickie #9
HIGHER ASSETS

Goal/results: Shape and strengthen your hamstrings and gluteal muscles (this time from a different angle than used in Fit Quickies #4, #5, and #10); strengthen the stabilizing postural muscles in your back; improve your posture in a convenient, travel-friendly, standing position

Workout time: Less than 5 minutes

Equipment: High-back chair, dance bar, countertop edge—or airport transit railing!

The Problem

Sitting for extended periods of time can lead to atrophy of the gluteal muscles due to constant pressure and lack of use. This, in turn, can contribute to low back pain and difficulty with some movements that naturally require the gluteal muscles to jump into action, such as standing up from a seated position, sitting down with control, and climbing stairs.

 If you were to track gluteal muscle activation via electromyography (EMG) for a day, chances are, you'd not detect a whole lot of action. That flat lining is what's giving us flat behinds.

Yet even if we are more active, the gluteals tend to be left behind in our workouts. We worked on weak, unconditioned, and shape-challenged glutes with Fit Quickies #4, #5, and #8. With the addition of Fit Quickie #9, I provide multiple opportunities and different angles in which you can engage those gorgeous gluteals and command them to take new shape.

The Facts

Gluteals and hamstrings should be exercised in a variety of ways and from a variety of angles. This includes large, compound muscle movement such as that found in squats and lunges. Targeted isolation work also has a place, especially if you're looking for some unique body shaping, as you're also doing with Fit Quickies #4 and #5.

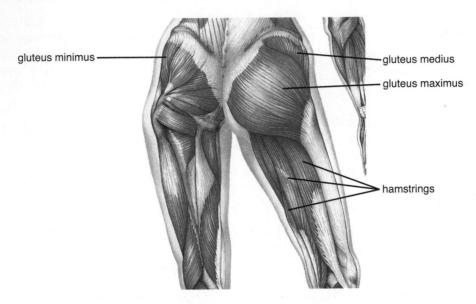

For best overall development of the multiple muscles through the back of your hips and thighs, challenge them from a variety of angles.

The Fit Quickie Fix

Do you need to get on the floor, on all fours, or perform a dramatic squat or lunge to challenge your gluteal and hamstring muscles? Not necessarily. For a quick—and very targeted, as you'll soon find out—alternative, you can work your backside while standing, anywhere and any time. How? By using Fit Quickie #9. As a matter of fact, look at this exercise as Fit Quickie #4 turned right side up, because that's exactly what it is, with a tweak or two.

Initially, I designed this exercise specifically to address travel concerns. I wanted the gluteal and hamstring shaping and strengthening I achieved with the on-the-floor Fit Quickies (#4, #5, and #8) but in a more convenient and portable standing position. So I turned the whole thing vertical and added some extra challenges with the setup—extra focus on pelvic position and specific attention to detail for the working leg.

This exercise has become a regular in my home workouts, and it will for you, too. It specifically targets your hamstrings and gluteals with the unique properties a standing position delivers. Because you're upright rather than horizontal, you get a whole new perspective on your glute and hamstring workload, with the added challenge of gravity the standing position brings.

As a bonus, this exercise also restores your posture through your entire body, all the way through your back and out the top of your head. Don't overlook your posture. It's all too easy to slump out of alignment when you're rushed, traveling, or simply on the go.

Yet with Fit Quickie #9, you can instantly align your standing posture and get an energy boost without any special equipment or the need to relocate. This makes it very convenient. I've done Fit Quickie #9 in airports, in parking lots, while waiting in supermarket lines, and while standing at my kitchen counter preparing dinner. It's a great quick pick-me-up whenever you need it.

 The gluteus maximus is a combination of fast-twitch and slow-twitch fibers. Fast-twitch fibers are tapped for power bursts, whereas the slow-twitchers are used during endurance activities, such as aerobic exercise. This means your gluteals benefit from both higher-load training with more resistance, as in Fit Quickie #12, and lower-load, higher-repetition exercises such as in Fit Quickie #9. Mix it up!

This exercise is specifically for lifting your seat by the way you position your body and isolate, target, and overload those muscles through the back of your body. Whenever you team up your gluteals and hamstrings, as you do here, the unique stacked positioning gives a whole lift to the entire area where the hamstrings and gluteals come into play. You'll love the uplifting result.

How to Do It

Think of Fit Quickie #9 as #4 in standing position. The setup is similar, but you'll feel the slight shift of focus.

Position

Here's your starting position:

1. Facing or on profile to your support, place your feet on the floor parallel, about 4 or 5 inches apart.

2. Soften your knees into a slight bend. This shouldn't be a deep knee bend; it should be just enough to drop your body a couple inches and allow you to complete the rest of the correct positioning.

3. Create the anchored neutral position you should now know well: pull in your abdominals and isometrically grip your gluteal muscles on both sides to anchor your pelvis, offsetting the tendency to release it into anterior tilt.

4. Line up your upper body correctly. Lift the weight of your ribs off your hips, lengthen your spine, open your chest, and have your shoulders back and anchored on your shoulder blades in back. Drop your shoulders down and away from your ears, and extend your energy out the top of your head to the ceiling. Your abdominals should be firm.

Check to be sure you're not leaning back. When you're vertical from your ears through your shoulder joint to your hips, you may feel like you're folding forward a little bit at the waist due to the light pelvic grip. Observe your alignment in a mirror if you need to until you get the feel of it. Your upper body will be straight up, although you're not aspiring to a flat back. Your spine will still demonstrate its natural curves.

Anchors

Here are your anchor points:

- Your feet on the floor

- Your tightened abdominal muscles

- Your gripped gluteal muscles and aligned pelvis

- Your shoulder blades locked on your rib cage in back

- Your fingertips placed lightly on your support

Isolate

From the slightly bent knee position, bend your right knee even more to pick your right foot off the floor, placing the toes of your right foot on the floor behind you. Keeping your left knee softly bent so your hips stay level, reconnect with your pelvis, pulling it back into alignment, and anchor it by isometrically gripping your glutes on both sides.

Bending your right knee even more, raise your right foot, and bring it up behind you toward your rear end without letting your right knee come forward past your left knee. Your right knee should be pointing almost straight to the ground, in a match with the position of your left knee. Bring your right foot up behind you as far as you can, while staying in good position, until you feel your hamstring "catch" and you're unable to lift it any farther—it'll feel as if it's butted up against your gluteals. Right away, you should feel your muscles struggle to hold you in position. That's a good thing.

Reconnect with the anchoring of your pelvis. You'll feel a stretch at the front of your hip where it joins your leg. Again, it's the fight to maintain correct position that powerfully engages the muscles you're isolating in this exercise. The isolation sets everything up for you beautifully—even before you begin the repetitions.

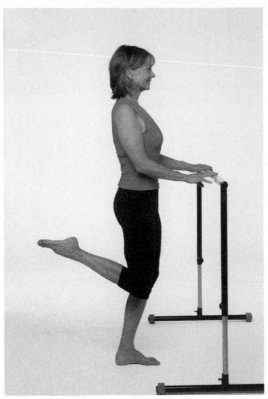

When you're in position, you'll feel the isolation and overload in your hamstrings and gluteals right away.

Repetitions

Here's how to do Fit Quickie #9:

1. Keeping your gluteals tight, pull your right heel up toward your rear end (1 second) and then lower your foot to touch your toes to the floor (1 second). Each "pull and touch" move should take about 2 seconds. This starts you off working your hamstring in its full range of motion before progressing to a tighter range. Keep your shoulders back and your abdominal muscles in and tight. Your hip joint should remain stretched open in front, and your right knee should point straight down to the floor. Your right knee will want to sneak forward so your gluteal muscles can get some relief from the work, but don't let it! Keep everything in place. You'll feel the intensity all the way up through the back of your leg and into your glutes. Do 8 repetitions.

2. Keeping your right knee bent with your right foot lifted behind you, pull the toes of your right foot toward the wall behind you by initiating a contraction from your gluteals. Take 1 second to pull your heel back, and hold for another second. Keep the grip in your glutes, keep your shoulders back and your posture lifted, and keep breathing. Do 8 repetitions. Each "pull and hold" should take about 2 seconds.

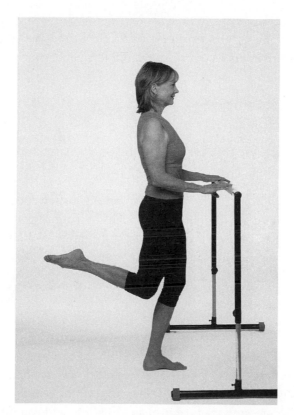

Note how my working leg is slightly behind my standing leg. This position alone deeply challenges your gluteals and hamstrings as you fight to maintain proper position through your entire upper body.

3. This is a combination of steps 1 and 2. Squeeze your heel in toward your glutes for 2 counts (as in step 1) and then press the toe of your right foot to the back wall by pulling from your gluteals, and hold (as in step 2). You're still isometrically gripped in the glutes of your standing leg as well. This should feel very challenging—that's how you change muscle. Squeeze, squeeze, pull, and hold for 8 repetitions. Each "squeeze, squeeze, pull, and hold" should take about 4 seconds

total: 1 second to squeeze once, 1 second to squeeze a second time, 1 second to press back, and 1 second in the hold position. Keep your hips level.

4. To finish, do 8 more pulls of your foot back, as in step 2, although now you're moving up tempo with one press-and-hold per second. Do 3 sets of 8 repetitions, for a total of 24.

Repeat with your left leg. Be sure to reconnect with your form: your glutes gripped with your pelvis tucked, your abdominals tight, your shoulders back, your rib cage lifted, and your spine long.

Stretch

Your mission is to complete Fit Quickie #9 standing, so you stretch your hamstrings and gluteals in a standing position, too:

1. To stretch your right leg, shift your weight onto your left foot and place the heel of your right foot on the floor about 12 inches in front of you. Even though you've shifted your weight, keep your hips square and aligned, avoiding the tendency to pop the hip of your standing leg out to the side.

2. Bend your left knee gently to allow your body to drop slightly downward, starting a forward fold at your hips.

3. Keeping your upper body strong and in good posture, with your chest open and your shoulder blades still anchored on your rib cage in back, continue to fold forward at your hips, pressing your chest forward over your extended right leg. Allow your rear end to extend and lift behind you rather than rounding over your extended leg. By pressing forward instead of pulling and rounding, you place the stretch exactly where you want it: on the back of your right leg and hip. Go right to the edge of the stretch, and breathe. As the muscles release, you'll be able to press farther into the stretch. Hold the stretch for 20 to 30 seconds.

Switch to the other side, and repeat.

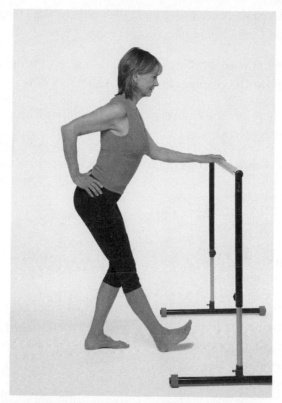

Move into the stretch slowly and mindfully to release your hamstring and gluteal muscles, which will be tight from the exercise. Lift your glutes to deepen the stretch.

Common Errors

Beware of these common errors while you exercise:

- During the exercise, don't lose connection with proper upper-body alignment. Don't lean back or round your shoulders forward as your body seeks to escape the work. Remember, fewer repetitions done well trumps many done with less focus, so stay mindful and line up correctly. Your body will repay you with optimal results.

- Don't let go of the contraction of your gluteals and your anchored pelvis as your muscles start to fatigue. If necessary, stop, reconnect with your anchors, and jump in again.

- Don't release the gluteals of your standing leg as your attention becomes preoccupied with your working leg.

- Don't let the heel of your working leg drop, releasing the contraction through your hamstrings.

- Don't grasp the support too vigorously to try to assist with the work of the exercise. Always keep a light touch!

- Don't sink into the hip of your standing leg. Keep your hips level.

Tips and Modifications

These tips and alternate ways to perform the exercise might help:

- During the repetition steps 2, 3, and 4, immediately following each "pull" of your heel either up or back toward the wall behind you, reanchor your pelvis with a curl under to deepen the gluteal contraction. This is a tiny move, but you'll feel the difference.

- If you experience any cramping in your hamstrings during the work phase, lower your foot closer to the floor and bring your attention back to the work in your gluteals. This is actually a powerful variation of this exercise, so keep that in mind.

- Alternate leading legs. Each time you do the exercise, start the work on a different side. This helps build muscle balance and keeps the challenge more unique, which is good news when it comes to creating muscle. Our bodies quickly adapt to any challenge, and by keeping things mixed up a little, you keep your body guessing and reap rewards in muscle shaping.

- To bring your inner thighs into the game, grip a rolled piece of foam (see Fit Quickie #4) between your legs, high up on your inner thighs. This helps keep your upper legs parallel as well.

To create even more intensity in Fit Quickie #9, you can rise onto the ball of the foot of your standing leg. This is known as *relevé* position in ballet. By coming up onto your foot this way, you immediately create a greater contraction through the back of your standing leg, from your calves all the way up through your gluteals. If you try this variation, be sure you are able to complete the basic version in good form first, before taking it a step further.

So there you have it—an excellent exercise for targeted body shaping you can use anytime, anywhere.

Fit Quickie #10
LEGS INTO PLAY

> **Goal/results:** Strengthen your calf muscles and stabilize your knee joints, stimulate movement of the lymphatic fluid through your lymph vessels, warm up and instantly invigorate your entire body
>
> **Workout time:** 2 minutes
>
> **Equipment:** High-back chair, dance bar, countertop edge—or airport transit railing!

The Problem

The calf muscles are largely underused and often out of play for several hours a day while we sit at desks and workstations, and in cars, trains, and airplanes. This has serious implications for your circulation. (More on this coming up.) The calves are also the first place you should get active when you need to warm up for exercise, stimulate circulation, or just plain get invigorated.

 Knee stability is largely a function of the soft tissues surrounding it—tendons, ligaments, and discs made of cartilage. These tissues form intricate connections and work as a team to stabilize your knee.

Perhaps your knees just aren't what they used to be. Maybe you're looking for a way to stabilize them without putting them into a compromising position. It's possible that even just the *thought* of bending your knees makes you wince. Although this might sound like a knee problem, don't forget that the muscles in your legs that run up to, down to, and through and around your knees play a complex role in the integrity of your knee joints. That includes your calf muscles, which is why calves and knees are worked together in this exercise.

The Facts

The knee is a very complex joint—and one we demand a lot of. Given that your knee is also smack dab in the middle of your longest limbs, your legs, you can see how it's susceptible to trouble.

Knee joint motion occurs in several directions and has multiple biomechanical functions. Take the simple act of walking, for instance. During the standing phase of walking, your knees stay slightly flexed to act as shock absorbers and to transmit forces through your lower legs. As your leg swings through on your stride, your knee flexes to shorten your leg so your foot can clear the ground on swing-through. The load on these functions becomes even heavier when you pick up the pace in a run.

Add to that the face that variations in knee alignment—from knock-knee to bow-leg and all points in between—are not uncommon, and you can see how you can easily encounter pain, injury, and other problems at the knee joints. And what about lateral movement demands, such as side-to-side action on the tennis or basketball court or the dance floor? Any way you put it, the stability challenges placed on your knees are enormous. No wonder knees are so susceptible to injury. Your knees need your tender loving care, and your calves are there to come to the rescue.

 Your knees employ an entire fleet of shock absorbers and friction reducers in the form of bursa sacks —14 of them!—and fat pads. Bursae release synovial fluid, a clear fluid secreted by membranes in joint cavities to lubricate the knee joint. Bursae can be injured by trauma, which leads to inflammation of the bursae called bursitis.

In addition, the flow of lymph from your legs toward your heart is the result of the pumping action of your calf muscles at work. This pumping action also circulates used blood from your lower legs up against gravity back to your upper body for refreshment and reoxygenation. In fact, the calf muscle is sometimes called the "peripheral heart" because of this important responsibility.

Also, as the muscles in your calves contract, lymph is squeezed out of your legs via your lymphatic vessels. Then, as your calf muscle relaxes, valves in the vessels shut, preventing the fluid from returning to your lower extremities. When you're inactive for periods of time, the whole circulation process slows down. No wonder you feel sluggish when you've been sitting for too long!

 Your lymphatic system works with your circulatory system to deliver nutrients, oxygen, and hormones from your blood to the cells that make up all the tissues of your body. This system also defends your body against disease by removing excess fluid, waste, debris, dead blood cells, pathogens, and toxins from both these cells and the tissue spaces between them. A sluggish lymphatic system is a sluggish immune system, and the fastest way to get the lymph fired up is to pump your calf muscles.

The Fit Quickie Fix

Fit Quickie #10 addresses several of these issues and delivers multiple payoffs for your calves and knees. This exercise, Legs into Play, is so named because it does just that—it brings all the muscles of your legs into play quite quickly and in a position that's ultrasafe and strengthening for your knees. It also stimulates your calf muscles and their very important functions.

Ten of your leg muscles cross or somehow come into play to stabilize your knee, and all of them jump into the game with this exercise—and in a knee-protective position. Because of this, Fit Quickie #10 is the ideal warm-up exercise to do before any other leg work that involves bending your knees. It also stands alone as an exercise, doubling as an instant energizer.

The superstar of the calf muscles, the gastrocnemius, runs from just above the knee down to the heel and is involved in standing, walking, running, and jumping. It's also the muscle that allows you to come high up onto the balls of your feet, as you do in Fit Quickie #10. No wonder this targeted exercise delivers such knee-stabilizing power.

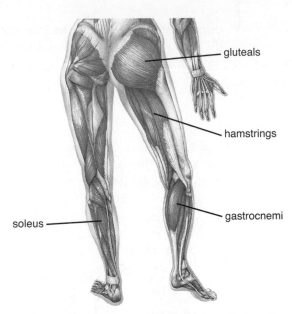

The muscles of the calves are multiple and many layered, including those that run through the knee as stabilizers.

Fit Quickie #10 also comes with some important bonus benefits. In addition to revving up your leg muscles and getting the fluids around your knee joints warmed and ready for action, you'll stimulate your lymphatic system. Legs into Play gets your lymph moving—fast.

How to Do It

This exercise is also one of the best instant invigorators you'll ever find. It's the perfect warm-up to sneak in before you do any of the lower-body Fit Quickies, such as #4, #5, #6, and #9.

Position 1

Legs into Play is done in 2 positions. Here's your starting position:

1. Stand facing or on profile to your support.

2. Place your feet parallel directly below your hips, 4 or 5 inches apart.

3. Get your upper body in correct alignment. Lift the weight of your ribs off your hips, lengthen your spine, open your chest, and have your shoulders back and anchored on your shoulder blades in back. Your abdominals should be firm, and your spine and pelvis should be in anchored position.

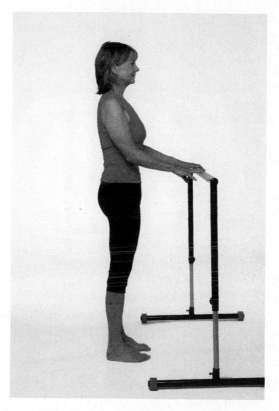

Feet placed, anchors engaged, and ready to go!

4. With the top of your head reaching toward the ceiling, and keeping your gluteals tightened to keep your pelvis in correct alignment, straighten your legs and use your calf muscles to rise up onto the balls of your feet.

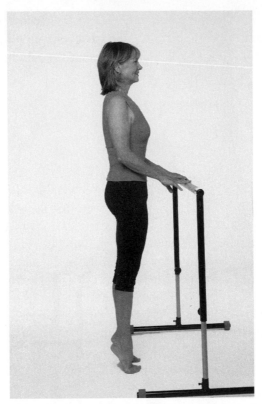

Rise onto the balls of your feet with a sharp contraction of your calf muscles. You should now feel all your muscles through your legs coming into play.

Anchors

Here are your anchor points:

- The balls of your feet on the floor

- Your hand lightly on your support

- Your shoulders anchored on your rib cage in back

- Your abdominals pulled in and your gluteals gripped to bring your pelvis into anchored position

Isolate

All the muscles of your legs and hips, both front and back, will be isometrically engaged and ready for action as soon as you rise up onto the balls of your feet.

Repetitions

Here's how Fit Quickie #10 works:

1. Keeping all the muscles in your glutes, thighs, and the backs of your legs isometrically contracted, and with your knees straight, tap your heels to the floor quickly 2 times and then rise up onto the balls of your feet again by sharply contracting your calf muscles. The 2 taps on the floor should take about 1 second, and rising up onto your toes and holding should take about 1 second. Do this 8 times.

2. Keeping your body in the same position as in step 1, tap your heels to the floor once instead of twice and then rise up onto the balls of your feet for 8 single-count repetitions. Each down-up cycle should take about 1 second.

Position 2

Place your feet flat on the floor, close together and touching. Keeping your heels together, pivot your feet outward from each other until you form a 90-degree angle at the point where your heels touch.

3. Repeat as in step 1 in this new, turned-out foot position.

4. Maintaining your same body position, tap your heels to the floor once and then rise up onto the balls of your feet for 16 repetitions. Each down-up cycle should take about 1 second.

By now, your blood will be pumping and your leg muscles will be warmed up. Whenever you work the large muscles in your legs, you get instantly energized. That's why I call this an instant invigorator.

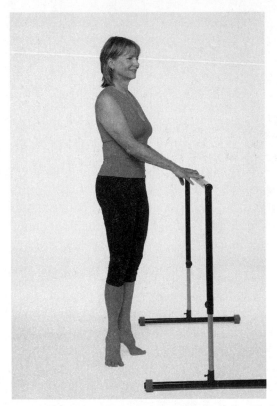

In position 2, your heels touch and your toes are turned out at a 90-degree angle.
Be sure the rest of your body is in line.

Stretch

Now for your well-deserved stretch:

1. Stand with both feet flat on the floor and parallel.

2. Step your right foot straight back behind you, about 2 or 3 feet. Be sure the toes of your back foot point straight ahead so you'll be stretching your right leg directly through the center of your calf muscles.

3. Keeping your upper body strong, gently lean forward toward your support while keeping your right heel pressed toward the floor. It's not important how far you go; what's important is feeling the stretch.

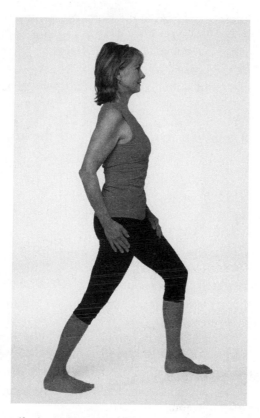

Follow the calf raises with a stretch. Be sure your toes are straight ahead
so you stretch right through the center of your calf.

4. Move right to the edge of the stretch, breathe, and hold for 20 to 30 seconds.

Repeat the stretch on your other leg.

Common Errors

Beware of these common errors while you exercise:

- Don't soften your knees and let go of the isometric contraction through your gluteals, hamstrings, and quadriceps muscles during the calf pumps. Keep everything active.

- Don't allow your pelvis and spine to slip out of proper alignment during the calf pumps.

- Don't let the toes of your back foot turn out during the stretch. Keep them pointing forward.

Tips and Modifications

These tips and alternate ways to perform the exercise might help:

- This exercise is so targeted, you'll feel it in your calves quite quickly. If finishing all the repetitions in correct form isn't possible, stop, do the stretch, and work your way up to more repetitions next time.

- Fit Quickie #10 is a must for airplane travel, as many health dangers are associated with sitting for extended periods of time, such as on a flight. In a pinch, you can even do this one sitting down in your airplane seat, working your calves from your bent knees down.

Legs into Play is my go-to choice for warm-up and instant invigoration in less than 2 minutes. Slip in this exercise before doing more demanding leg exercises to be sure your knees and leg muscles are ready for action.

Fit Quickie #11
UPPER-BODY SOS

Goal/results: Strengthen the muscles of your upper body and core; lift your bust line; improve your posture; improve your shoulder stability

Workout time: Less than 4 minutes

Equipment: None

The Problem

Collapsed posture, rounded shoulders, a sunken chest, shape-free arms, and droopy pectorals and their surrounding tissues—these are all signs of an upper body that lacks strength. Loss of upper-body strength also translates to a diminished ability to keep up with the demands of daily living.

The Facts

Each task you give your arms, shoulders, and back demands upper-body strength. When these upper-body muscles are weak, you're more prone to aches, pains, and injuries. And without some solid muscle attached to your bones, your upper-body posture and shape will continue to deteriorate.

Unlike your legs, which carry the weight of your entire body, your chest, shoulders, and arms are minimally challenged, and extra resistance is required to give them a push to be stronger. The best protection is to strengthen your upper-body muscles, and specific exercises for these muscles are essential. This is where push-ups and planks come in.

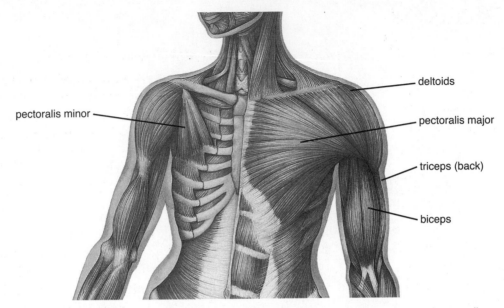

- deltoids
- pectoralis major
- triceps (back)
- biceps
- pectoralis minor

Fit Quickie #11 challenges the largest muscles on the front of your upper body, your pectorals, as well as your shoulders, arms, and core.

Push-ups are the best way to build overall upper-body strength. As a multijoint exercise, they use several of your joints and muscles simultaneously. They work not only your chest, but also your arms, including your triceps; your shoulders; and your midsection as a whole. Push-ups are an ultra-efficient, portable exercise that target many muscles quickly, and all at once.

Planks are also a multijoint exercise, although they're isometric. Planks can make many of the same strength claims to fame as push-ups. They offer a little variety, can be a safer place to start, and bring unrivaled challenge to the abdominals and all the other muscles of the core. As a matter of fact, many physical therapists use planks with clients as their first go-to move for building core strength and preventing back pain because of their superior ability to recruit the transversus abdominus muscle.

Consider push-ups and planks a dynamic duo you can—and should—mix up, alternate, or otherwise regularly work into your exercise rotation.

The Fit Quickie Fix

Push-ups and planks may not be the newest or most creative exercises on the block, but I consider these tried-and-true, no-special-equipment-required exercises necessary in any workout arsenal. I want you doing both of these strength- and shape-builders over the course of the week as your ability allows. If push-ups are too much of a strength reach for you just now, or if you have specific shoulder limitations, planks can be a great tool to help you work your way up. They're a powerhouse move on their own.

First we look at a few specifics about push-ups and then we move on to planks.

Push-ups confession: for a long time, I avoided doing them. I'm not going to kid you—push-ups are tough. However, this exercise is the best at strengthening the pectoral muscles of your chest and also your shoulders, as well as shaping the muscles in your arms, strengthening your core muscles, and lifting your bust line. For these reasons, I've made push-ups a mainstay in my workouts for the past several years. Do I like them any more than I used to? No. Do I find they deliver like no other upper-body challenge out there? Yes.

If you want more mobility and a stronger body that gets you through the day with vitality and gusto to spare, you need to master the push-up. And mastery involves nothing more than regular practice.

How to Do It

Although push-ups are one of the most basic of exercises, they're often done ineffectively. The key to success in this exercise—and, by now, this should sound familiar—is correct form. Success also demands that you select a variation best suited for your current ability level. That way, you'll be able to complete this exercise safely and effectively, and you'll enjoy big changes in the strength and shape of your upper body.

If it's been some time since you did your last push-up, or if you have shoulder issues—which must be respected—start with the bent-knee version.

Position: Bent-Knee Push-Ups

Here's your starting position:

1. Start in a quadruped position on the floor, on your hands and knees with your hands directly under your shoulders about shoulder width apart. Place your knees right beneath your hips, and position your thumbs almost directly beneath your shoulders. Think "on all fours."

2. Engaging the muscles deep in your abdomen, and keeping your knees bent to the 90-degree angle from your setup position on all fours, walk your hands forward approximately 6 inches and grip your gluteals enough to slightly tilt the top of your pelvis back. This anchors your body, putting you into safe, back-protective position with all your core muscles fired up.

3. Keep your head and neck in alignment with the rest of your body so you have a straight line from your ears through your shoulders to your knees.

4. Drop your shoulders down from your ears, and lock your shoulder blades onto your rib cage in back.

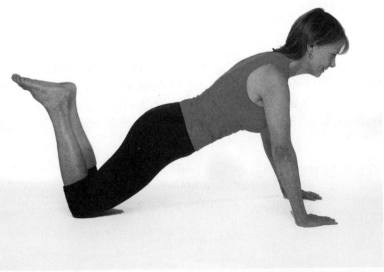

Before your first repetition, be sure you're hitting all your anchor points for stabilization.

Anchors

Here are your anchor points:

- Your hands and knees on the floor

- Your gripped gluteal muscles

- Your abdominal muscles, braced and ready, with your pelvis anchored

- Your shoulder blades locked onto your rib cage in back

Isolate

With all your anchors in place, bend your elbows slightly to bring the muscles of your chest and arms into play. You now have everything engaged and ready to go.

Repetitions

Here's what to do:

1. Inhale and bend your elbows to lower your body—while keeping your back straight—until your chest (not your head) is about 4 inches from the floor. Be sure to only lower as much as you can while keeping good form through your shoulders and back.

2. Exhale, engage your abdominals again (remember how from Fit Quickie #1?), and push the floor away until your arms are straight although not locked at the elbow. Keep your chest open, with your shoulder blades back in position to protect your shoulder joint. Keep your gluteals contracted throughout the push away from the floor.

Practice 10 to 15 repetitions, rest 15 seconds, and complete 1 or 2 more sets. Your ultimate goal is to be able to complete 2 sets of 12 to 20 repetitions, or 1 set of about 30 repetitions, in good form.

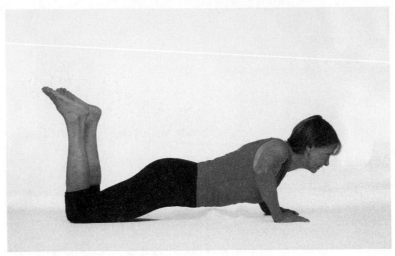

Bent-knee push-ups are your starting point for building good form and strength in push-ups.

Form trumps reps! Remember, correct alignment is far more important than high numbers of repetitions. This is true of push-ups just as much as (if not more than) other exercises. If you can do only 1 set of 3 repetitions in good form, that's exactly where you should start. You'll be able to work your way up by adding more sets and repetitions. Remember, safety first!

Position: Straight-Leg Push-Ups

Here's your starting position:

1. Get yourself into the same position as with bent-knee push-ups (steps 1 through 4).

2. Walk your right foot and then your left foot backward until your knees are straight and your body forms a line from your ankles through your hips to your shoulders. Avoid either drooping your head or looking up to the ceiling; let your neck be in a natural curve with either your gaze slightly forward or your chin gently tucked into your neck.

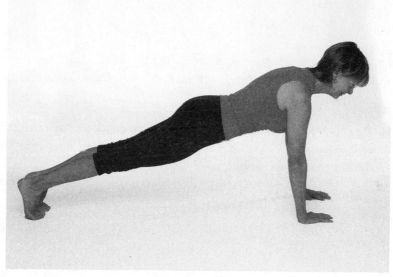

Straight-leg push-ups require a greater level of strength than bent-knee push-ups. Maintain your alignment as you lower your chest toward the floor.

Anchors

Here are your anchor points:

- Your hands and toes on the floor

- Your gripped gluteal muscles

- Your abdominal muscles, braced and ready, with your pelvis anchored

- Your shoulder blades locked onto your rib cage in back

Isolate

When you're in starting position, you've already isolated and engaged the muscles of your chest, shoulders, arms, and core.

Repetitions

Here's what to do:

1. Inhale and bend your elbows—while keeping your back straight—until your chest (not your head) is about 4 inches from the floor. As in bent-knee pushups, go no lower than you can with proper form.

2. Exhale, engage your abdominals again, and push the floor away until your arms are straight, although not locked at the elbow. Keep your chest open, with your shoulder blades back in position, to protect your shoulder joint.

Practice 10 to 15 repetitions, rest 15 seconds, and complete 2 more sets. Your ultimate goal is to be able to complete 2 sets of 12 to 20 repetitions or 1 set of about 30 repetitions in good form.

 If you're able to complete only a couple straight-leg push-ups, you can start there and move immediately into position for bent-knee push-ups by dropping your knees to the floor. Reconnect with your alignment before going on, and do as many bent-knee push-ups as you can to finish. This way, you'll gradually be able to increase your repetitions of straight-leg push-ups.

Position: Planks

Planks have an extraordinary ability to flatten the abdomen, relieve back pain, strengthen the core from abdominal muscles to the gluteals, and restore power to the upper body. In other words, watch out chest, shoulders, and arms—you're about to get a workout!

1. As in push-ups, start in a quadruped position on the floor.

2. Drop to your elbows, which should now be directly under your shoulders, to where your hands just were, creating a 90-degree bend at your elbows. Keep your forearms extended straight forward on the floor from your elbows.

Don't grasp your hands together because this activates your latissimus dorsi—the large muscle in your back—and brings them into the game. That's not a bad thing necessarily, but you're trying to keep the workload in your arms, shoulders, pectorals, and abdominal wall.

3. Walk your right foot and then your left foot backward until your knees are straightened and your body forms a line from your ears through your hips and shoulders and to your ankles. Avoid either drooping your head or looking up to the ceiling; let your neck be in a natural curve with either your gaze slightly forward or your chin gently tucked into your neck.

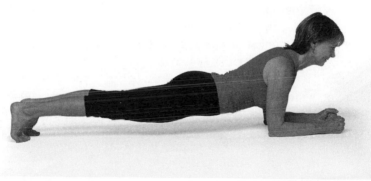

Planks are a superior standalone upper- and full-body strengthener and can be a very effective stepping stone to push-ups.

Anchors

Here are your anchor points:

- Your elbows, hands, and toes on the floor

- Your gripped gluteal muscles

- Your abdominal muscles, braced and ready, with your pelvis anchored

- Your shoulder blades locked onto your rib cage in back

Isolate

Once you walk your feet out in planks, your whole body will get busy with muscle activation to maintain your position.

Repetitions

The plank is measured by time held in position rather than reps. Start with a 10-second hold, rest for 15 seconds, and repeat. If 10-second holds are easy, progress to 15-second holds and work your way up to two 30-second holds with a 15-second rest in between, or one 45- to 60-second hold.

Stretch

To stretch the muscles of your chest, stand in a doorway and make a T with your upper arms. Then bend your elbows so you're in "goalpost" position. Place your forearms against the door frame and step or lean forward gently until you feel a stretch. Hold for 30 seconds and then relax.

If the door frame is too wide, stretch one side at a time. Place one forearm against the door frame, with your elbow bent, and turn your upper body away from the door frame as you stretch your arm. Hold for 30 seconds, and repeat with the other arm.

Variation: Knee Planks

You can practice planks on your knees, too. Simply drop your knees to the floor from straight-leg plank position. This is an excellent starting point from which to work your way up.

Common Errors

Beware of these common errors while you exercise:

- Don't launch into push-ups or planks without first engaging the muscles of your hips, abdominals, and cervical spine as anchors.

- Don't let your shoulders creep up toward your ears or let your back curve out of position as your body fights to keep form—this applies to both exercises. Be sure to keep your shoulders pulled down from your ears and watch for the tendency to round your upper back—it's another way your body will try to relieve the workload through the middle of your body.

- Don't let your head droop or extend your chin forward. Both can place a strain on your neck.

- Don't hold your breath during either exercise. Keep breathing throughout.

Tips and Modifications

These tips and alternate ways to perform the exercise might help:

- A shoulder injury, surgery, or otherwise compromised shoulder joint may prevent you from completing "regular" push-ups safely. This is no cause for shame. In fact, I've seen many who are proud of their "real" push-ups lower their chest only halfway to the floor. If your push-up is still in "half-court," so to speak, you're better off dropping to your knees and working a fuller range of motion. The important thing is getting your upper body challenged.

- You don't need to go all the way to the ground when doing push-ups to make them effective. As soon as your hips start sagging or your back starts rounding, your repetitions for that round are over. That's the point from where you work your way up.

- If you experience discomfort in your wrists while doing push-ups, you can use grip handles or grasp dumbbells instead of placing your hands directly on the floor. This reduces the amount of stress on your joints.

- If you're unable to keep correct alignment with either the push-ups or planks on your toes or on your knees, do wall push-ups or planks in a standing position instead. Simply take all the setup instructions for push-ups or planks to the wall. Walk your feet a distance back from the wall to create your plank.

- If you're new to planks or simply need a refresher course on proper form, you can practice the plank position—unloaded—in standing position.

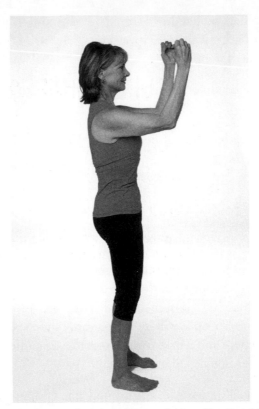

You can practice correct plank form in an upright position first. Line up your anchors, elbows, shoulders, and neckline while standing.

Practice push-ups and planks about three times a week to make sure and steady progress strengthening and shaping your upper body. Of all the moves you can add to your exercise routines, these come with so many bonus advantages, they may just be able to claim "We're number 1!" in the workout world.

Fit Quickie #12
SUPER-SHAPER SPLIT SQUATS

Goal/results: Strengthen and shape your entire lower body, building better gluteals and thighs, including your inner thighs

Workout time: 4 minutes

Equipment: Beginner: high-back chair, dance bar, countertop edge; intermediate/advanced: pair of dumbbells

The Problem

Underdeveloped gluteals, hamstrings, quadriceps, and even inner thighs result in weak lower-body strength, shape, and stability, as well as poor agility. This leads to reduced overall balance, shape, and gusto.

Agility is the ability to move quickly and easily—think nimble. The compound movements of Fit Quickie #12 build agility and functional gait, or the way you walk, step, and stride.

In addition to the isolation and overload work you've learned for these muscles in Fit Quickies #2, #4, #5, #6, #8, and #9, including exercises that work several big, important muscles at once, this one is a powerful addition to your strength and body-shaping plan. There's a reason I've named the split squat a "super shaper."

The Facts

Squats come in all flavors and long have been a gym standard. The split squat, a carryover from leg power-up routines I did in dance class and during my days as a gym rat, is my favorite version. You can count on my Fit Quickie tweaks to make this exercise safe and effective, whether you're a beginner or are more advanced and need a tune-up on this classic exercise.

The split squat requires a certain amount of coordination, some lower-body strength, and healthy knees. If you're a beginner to exercise, work your way up to this one after you've gained some initial strength and coordination with other lower-body Fit Quickies.

The Fit Quickie Fix

The split squat is a multijoint, compound exercise. It works your legs and hips, but your quadriceps—the muscles on the front of your thigh—are the prime mover. Many exercises work this muscle, but the split squat does so in a balanced manner, activating all four muscles of your quadriceps in a ratio superior to many other exercises. Your hamstrings and gluteals function to stabilize your knees and hips during the exercise, and your gluteus maximus helps straighten your thigh as you stand.

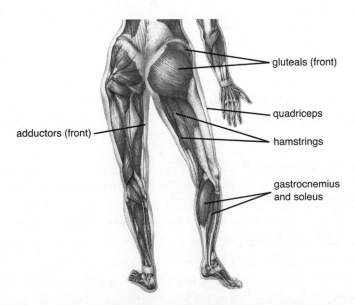

The split squat works your inner thighs, the fronts and backs of your thighs, your hips, and your calves in concert, challenging your balance as well as your musculature.

Your hip joints, knees, and ankles join forces with all the muscles in your legs and hips to execute this superior body shaper. This exercise targets the entire group so you have all those lower-body muscles in play, together, in a fast and effective manner.

How to Do It

With this exercise, you start in standing position, lower one knee toward the floor in the split squat, and push your feet into the floor to bring yourself back to a standing position.

Position

Here's your starting position:

1. Stand with your feet parallel directly below your hips, about 4 or 5 inches apart. Beginners should have a chair, counter, or bar at their side to provide stability and balance as you learn the exercise. You want to be able to feel this in the muscles you're targeting, without worrying about your balance as you get acquainted with this move. Intermediate exercisers: have your hands on your waist or your arms at your sides. Advanced exercisers: hold a dumbbell in each hand. Always start light and work your way up.

2. Connect with your proper form by getting your body lined up. Lift the weight of your ribs off your hips, lengthen your spine, open your chest, and have your shoulders back, with your shoulder blades anchored on your rib cage in back. Your abdominals should be firm, and your spine and pelvis should be anchored in neutral position.

3. Step your left foot straight back about 2½ feet, depending on the length of your legs, and place the ball of your left foot into position on the floor. Your left foot should be far enough back that, when you drop into the low position, your body weight doesn't pitch you forward or take your weight off the heel of your right front foot. Your front foot will stay flat on the floor. Notice that as you extend your left leg behind you, your pelvis is going to move into a slight anterior tilt. This is correct position; at the same time, your job is to keep your abdominal muscles active and your gluteals engaged to provide support through your spine.

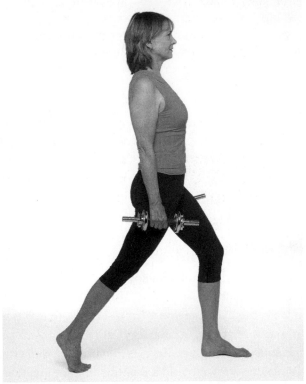

Line up everything carefully before lowering straight down into the split squat.

Anchors

Here are your anchor points:

- Your feet on the floor—the heel of your front foot and the ball of your back foot

- Your hand lightly on your support, on your waist, or lightly grasping the dumbbells (depending on the version you're doing)

- Your abdominals braced

- Your shoulders anchored on your rib cage in back

- Your gluteals gripped to offset excessive anterior pelvic tilt

Isolate

Keeping the toes of both feet straight ahead, soften your back knee slightly. This creates the downward movement of your upper body. Pause here to contract your abdominal muscles, pulling your belly button into your spine and contract your glutes to help you hold position through your pelvis. Feel the weight of your body on the heel of your front foot at all times. So when starting with your left leg back and your right foot in front, feel your weight in your right heel.

You should feel your leg and gluteal muscles engage.

Repetitions

Here's how it works:

1. Keeping your shoulders and hips lined up and your pelvis anchored, drop your hips straight downward by bending your knees, keeping the knee of your front leg directly over your toes in front. Drop as far down as you can without pitching your upper body forward, taking the weight off your front heel, or compromising your front knee. Take 3 seconds to lower your back knee toward the floor in a controlled fashion.

2. Drive your front heel and the ball of your back foot into the floor, squeeze your gluteals, and power your body back up into starting position.

Completing a cycle of step 1 and step 2 is one repetition. You want to work your way up to a set of 10 to 15 repetitions. Rest 15 seconds and do a set on the other leg. The minute you find yourself compromising your form, stop. Beginners: start with one set on each side. Intermediate and advanced: rest 15 seconds and do another set on each side.

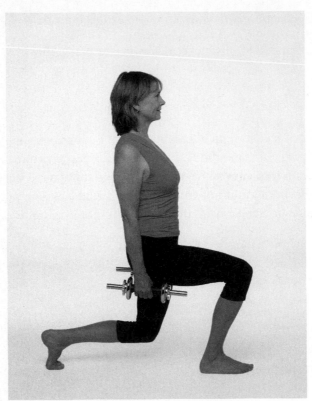

Deliberately move into the low position, yet come down only as far as you can while maintaining good form.

Stretch

Follow this exercise with the standing hamstring stretch as in Fit Quickie #9, as well as the quadriceps stretch from Fit Quickie #6.

Common Errors

Beware of these common errors while you exercise:

- Don't progress too quickly to a level your strength, knees, and stability may not be prepared for. Be sure to work your way up to safe proficiency with how low you move into the squat and how much weight you add as resistance. Using your body weight alone provides plenty of challenge as you get started.

- Don't allow your shoulders to fall forward of your hips. Be sure you have a vertical drop when moving down into the squat.

- Don't allow your weight to come off your heel in front, pitching your upper body farther forward and compromising your knee. At no point should the knee of your front leg move farther forward than the ends of your toes. If you're only lowering into a half-squat position, your knee will move no farther forward than the ankle of your front foot.

- Don't allow your front knee to roll in toward the midline of your body. Your front knee should stay straight, forward in the direction of the toes of your front foot.

- Don't allow your pelvis to tilt too far forward into excessive anterior pelvic tilt. Keep your pelvis anchored throughout the move by engaging your abdominals, and offset the tendency of your tail to pop back as you drop into the squat by keeping your glutes gripped and your tail tucked under.

Tips and Modifications

These tips and alternate ways to perform the exercise might help:

- Descend into the low position only as far as you can in proper alignment and form. If that's only 1 or 2 inches down from standing position, so be it! This is *the* way to prevent injury and build strength.

- If you're new to this exercise or haven't done it for some time, have a support at your side. That way, you can get a feel for the exercise, track your joints properly, and also become aware of the muscles you're working. You should feel it in your thighs and glutes. Your balance should feel challenged as well.

- When you feel like you've figured out the move with the help of a support, you can try it without the support.

- When you've mastered the move with no support and can complete the full range of motion with your back knee hovering within inches of the floor, you can start to add light handheld weights.

- When you've mastered the basics of this exercise, you can vary the speed of your descent into the squat and the drive back to standing. Keep your muscles guessing!

The stronger you get with this exercise and the more stable your front knee, the bigger the range of motion you can challenge yourself with—up to an approximate 90-degree angle in your back knee. Not everyone can do this, however, so respect your own limitations.

And don't be surprised if you feel this one in your inner thighs the next day. Remember, your leg adductors are stabilizers, and they are called upon more than you might suspect with this move. That's part of what makes it such a keeper!

Fit Quickie #13
BACK BEAUTY

> **Goal/results:** Strengthen the muscles of your upper back and the backs of your shoulders to create beautiful posture, alleviate neck and back pain, stabilize your shoulder joints, and increase upper-body vitality
>
> **Workout time:** Less than 4 minutes
>
> **Equipment:** Large stability ball or physioball

The Problem

Rounded shoulders are epidemic these days when we spend so much time seated. Focusing down and forward with our upper bodies is reflected in poor posture, rounded shoulders, a weak upper back, and a slouchy upper body. This leads to upper-back and neck pain, neck vertebrae and shoulder joint impingement, a forward head, and poor movement patterns. Without specifically countering the forward slouch and unconditioned muscles of the upper back and backs of shoulders, you're looking at chronic neck and back pain, shoulder issues, and hump-backed posture.

This is compounded by the fact that your shoulders are a very fragile joint you place complex demands on. They must be mobile enough for everything you do using your arms and hands, yet they also must be stable enough to allow for all the lifting, pushing, and pulling actions you perform during the course of the day. It's easy to see why this compromise between mobility and stability results in a large number of shoulder issues. Neck tension combined with frequent overhead loading, as when you reach your arms above your head, exacerbates the problem.

The Facts

About 80 percent of us will experience back pain at some time in our lives, and most of it is preventable. Improving the strength of your upper back and also the health of your shoulder joint dramatically improves your physical carriage, strength, and odds of living free from shoulder pain.

 If you tend to sit in a slumped position, the muscles of your upper and middle back become overstretched and weak. This predisposes you to a long list of neck and shoulder problems. Time to straighten up!

The Fit Quickie Fix

"Back beauty" is my catch phrase for the two big-time exercises featured in Fit Quickie #13. Straight from physical therapy exercises, these moves are known as Ys and Ts, so named because of the way you position your body for the exercises. These exercises work the complex network of muscles in your upper back, along with the muscles at the backs of your shoulders, including the rhomboids and the upper, middle, and lower trapezius muscles. These muscles all insert on the scapula, your shoulder blades. Proper movement and strength of the scapula is essential for shoulder injury prevention—and for a functional and beautiful upper back.

Luckily, these muscles are easy to isolate and challenge— yielding rapid results. Fit Quickie #13 helps improve your posture and the health of your shoulder joints, which tie into the rest of your torso; the foundation of a healthy, strong upper back; and the carriage of physical confidence.

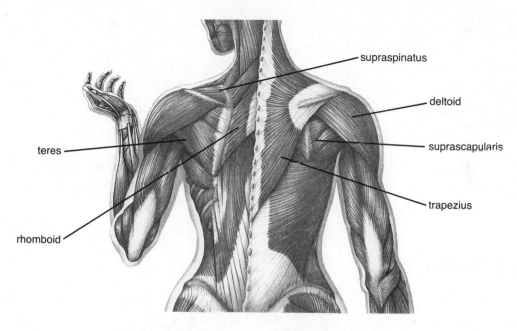

The muscles of the upper back and backs of the shoulders.

How to Do It

You'll need a physioball for to support your body for this exercise. Physioballs come in many sizes. Most will work well here.

Position: Ys

Here's your starting position for Ys:

1. Support your weight on top of the physioball, keeping your head and neck in alignment with the rest of your body so you have a fairly straight line from your ears through your spine, and you have a strong line from your head to your toes. Depending on the size of the ball, you may have a slight forward bend at your hips, although you should still be able to keep your spine correctly aligned straight from your hips through your shoulders. Grip the floor with your toes.

2. Engage your abdominals and slightly tuck your pelvis into neutral position to stabilize your body on the ball.

3. Straighten your arms and extend them to form a Y forward of your upper body, with your thumbs pointing toward the ceiling and the outside of your hands resting on the floor.

Your thumbs are up on these exercises to create a rotation of your arm that allows you to avoid impingement of your shoulder joint.

4. Press your shoulders down from your ears and anchor your shoulder blades on your rib cage in back.

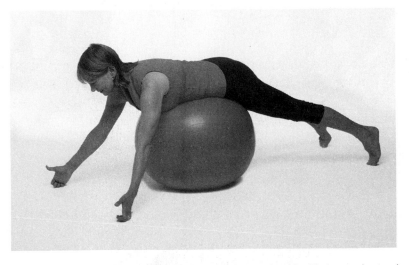

To begin the Ys, anchor your body on the physioball, secure your shoulder blades, and extend your arms in a Y in front of you on the floor.

Anchors

Here are your anchor points:

- Your toes on the floor

- Your abdominal muscles, braced and ready

- Your gripped gluteal muscles, in pelvic anchor

- Your shoulders down from your ears

- Your shoulder blades locked on your rib cage in back

Isolate

Squeeze your shoulder blades together to lift your hands off the floor in front of you. You've now just isolated and overloaded the network of muscles in your upper back and the backs of your shoulders.

Repetitions

Here's what to do:

1. Anchoring your shoulder blades toward each other on your back, lift your arms off the floor until they're extended into a Y straight forward from your back. Don't bring your arms higher than your back; that puts undue pressure on your shoulder joint capsule.

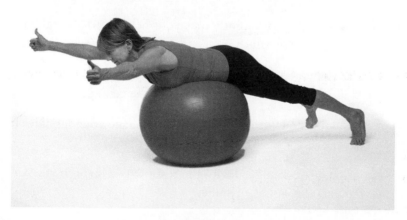

Bring your arms up only until they're level with your back to avoid taxing your shoulder joint.

2. With control, lower your hands to the floor again, keeping your thumbs up and your shoulders pressed down and away from your ears.

Practice 10 to 15 repetitions, rest 15 seconds, and complete another set. Your ultimate goal is to be able to complete 2 sets of 15 repetitions in good form.

 If you're a beginner, your range of motion for these exercises may be smaller than a more experienced exerciser would have. That doesn't matter; challenging your muscles is what counts! Your range of motion will improve as you gain strength and flexibility.

Position: Ts

Here's your starting position for Ts:

1. Support your weight right on top of the physioball, keeping your head and neck in alignment with the rest of your body so you have a straight line from your ears through your spine and you have a strong line from your head to your toes. Depending on the size of the ball, you may have a slight forward bend at your hips, although you should still be able to keep your spine correctly aligned from your hips through your shoulders. Grip the floor with your toes.

2. Engage your abdominals and slightly tuck your pelvis into neutral position to stabilize your body on the ball.

3. Extend your straightened arms to form a T, with your arms reaching out to the sides of your body and your thumbs pointing toward the ceiling.

4. Press your shoulders down from your ears, and engage your shoulder blades on your rib cage in back.

5. Keep your head and neck aligned with the rest of your body so you have a straight line from your ears through your spine.

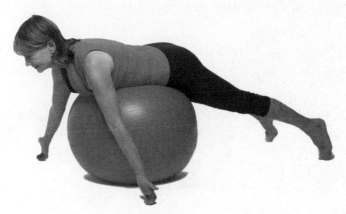

Reconnect with all your anchor points, and glide your shoulder blades in toward each other before beginning.

Anchors

Your anchors are the same as for the Ys.

Isolate

Once in starting position, you've already isolated and engaged the muscles of your chest, shoulders, and arms.

Repetitions

Here's what to do:

1. Anchoring your shoulder blades toward each other on your back, lift your arms off the floor until they're extended into a T straight out to your sides. Do not let your arms go higher than your back, to avoid impinging upon your shoulder joint.

2. With control, lower your hands to the floor again, keeping your thumbs up and your shoulders pressed down and away from your ears.

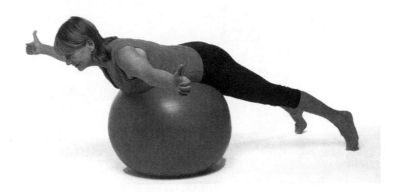

With Ts, you raise your arms directly to the side.

Practice 10 to 15 repetitions, rest 15 seconds, and complete another set. Your ultimate goal is to be able to complete 2 sets of 15 repetitions in good form.

 Transfer the shoulder-placement skills you're learning with the Ys and Ts to other activities and exercises. Every time you raise your arms overhead is an opportunity to practice correct anchoring of your shoulder, down and away from your ears.

Stretch

Now to stretch the muscles of your upper back and the backs of your shoulders:

1. Sit cross-legged on the floor, and lace your fingers together in front of you. Invert your palms by turning your thumbs in toward you and then down.

2. Gently extend your arms forward. You'll feel the stretch in the backs of your shoulders and in all the muscles of your upper back. Hold the stretch for 30 seconds.

During the stretch, breathe deeply, expanding your rib cage and stretching your back from the inside, with your expanding lungs pressing outward.

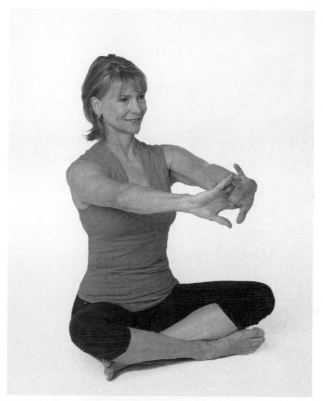

Take your time with the stretch! Keep your shoulders down from your ears and imagine you're breathing into your back.

Variation

When you can easily accomplish 2 sets of 15 reps with each exercise, you can add more resistance with dumbbells. Start with no more than a 1-pound dumbbell in each hand. Be sure to keep the correct position of rotation at your wrists, with the thumb side of your hands toward the ceiling. When you add more resistance, it may become necessary to decrease the number of repetitions at first.

Common Errors

Beware of these common errors while you exercise:

- Don't completely let go of the engagement in your muscles anchoring your scapula in back. Your shoulder blades will slide in toward each other and then move apart somewhat during the course of the exercise. As they tire, you'll be inclined to let them go. When this happens, stop, rest, and begin your next set. You'll increase your repetitions quickly with regular practice.

- Don't let your shoulders creep up to your ears as the muscles in your back and the backs of your shoulders tire. Keep lots of space between your ears and your shoulders. If your shoulders start to sneak up toward your ears, stop your repetitions and rest.

- Don't let your head droop or extend your chin forward and tilt your head up. Doing so can place a strain on your neck.

Tips and Modifications

These tips and alternate ways to perform the exercise might help:

- If you don't have a physioball, you can use an exercise bench or other similar platform. Even a step aerobics platform will work in a pinch. Do not, however, do these flat on the floor. Your range of motion will be too limited, and raising your arms into the Y or T will require you to overextend your shoulder joint.

- These look and feel easy as you get started, yet after a few repetitions, you'll discover how challenging they really are—and their great potential for building a beautiful back and posture.

Don't be fooled by the seeming simplicity of these exercises. They're the first thing a physical therapist pulls out of his or her bag of tricks when it comes to restoring shoulder strength and mobility. You'll be surprised at how quickly you feel your muscles at work, and equally pleased with the changes these two gems make in your upper-body posture and alignment as they strengthen the muscles of your upper back and the back of your shoulders.

Fit Quickie #14
SHOULDER SHAPERS

Goal/results: Shape and strengthen the muscles of your shoulders

Workout time: Less than 3 minutes

Equipment: 1- to 6-pound dumbbells

The Problem

Weak shoulder muscles and muscle imbalance can mean an upper body that's prone to injury. This undercuts upper-body function, making those bags of groceries, for example, harder to lift. Unchallenged shoulder muscles lose shape and size, set you up for shoulder injury, and make your shoulder carriage and entire upper body look—and feel—feeble.

I bet you know someone—probably more than one person—who has suffered a shoulder injury, from rotator cuff to frozen shoulder, to soft shoulder tissues, causing pain and inflammation. Or perhaps you have experienced one of these debilitating injuries yourself.

The Facts

Your shoulder muscles work with your entire shoulder joint and your shoulder blade to move your arms forward, backward, and sideways. Add to this the motions of your arms over as well as behind your head and back, and you can easily see the potential for shoulder injury.

Like your hip joint, your shoulder is a ball-and-socket joint. It's the most mobile joint in your body, answering all the demands you place on it in so many different directions. At the same time, your shoulder socket is small and relatively shallow, which tremendously compromises its stabilizing function. To compensate, a network of ligaments and muscles surrounds and supports your shoulder. These soft tissues work together to hold the joint in place.

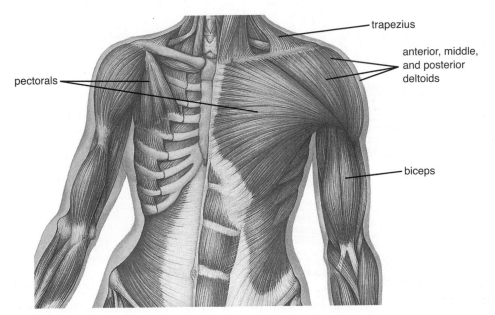

Your shoulder muscles support a wide range of motions and movements for such a relatively small joint.

If any of these ligaments and muscles gets weak, strained, sprained, or just fatigued, the ball and socket can slip out of alignment, resulting in a number of very uncomfortable conditions. It may start with instability of your shoulder and lead to joint dislocation, which is extremely painful. It can also be a precursor to more serious injuries of the shoulder, such as shoulder impingement or full-blown rotator cuff injuries. Impingement is caused by the acromion bone of the shoulder repeatedly coming into contact with the shoulder muscles as you raise your arm. If not addressed or treated, this can lead to tears in the soft tissue and rotator cuff injuries.

So you never want to just "work through" shoulder discomfort or tightness. With the stress your shoulders endure, strengthening and flexibility exercises are crucial for keeping them healthy and beautiful.

If you have had a shoulder injury or a history of shoulder issues, you know how important it is to keep your shoulders in shape. I designed Fit Quickie #14 with the utmost safety in mind, avoiding overhead arm movements that put your shoulders in a potentially compromising position.

The Fit Quickie Fix

Fit Quickie #14 asks you first to anchor your shoulder joint into a fully functional, aligned, and safe position. Then you deliberately lift resistance to strengthen and shape the front of your shoulders, all without compromising your shoulder joint as you would by lifting a weight over your head.

In concert with push-ups and Fit Quickie #13, you'll have a robust shoulder challenge and stability program.

How to Do It

You can do this exercise kneeling, sitting, or standing. Let's start with the kneeling position, although if kneeling presents a problem for your knees, you can easily substitute a seating or standing position.

Position

Here's your starting position:

1. Kneel on the floor, on one knee, in "marriage proposal" position.

2. Place your upper body in proper alignment, as you do for the standing Fit Quickies. Upright your spine so the weight of your ribs is lifted from your ribs and your shoulders are stacked over your hips. Open your chest, and secure your position by engaging the muscles through your mid- and upper back to stabilize your upper-body posture. Wrap your shoulder blades securely around your rib cage in back. Firm your abdominal muscles, and anchor your pelvis.

3. Extend the crown of your head to the ceiling, and drop your shoulders from your ears, creating length in your neck.

4. Bend your elbows to 90 degrees at your waist. Beginners: don't use any added weight while you get the idea of the exercise. Then add 1- or 2-pound weights. You can eventually work up to 5- or 6-pound weights in each hand.

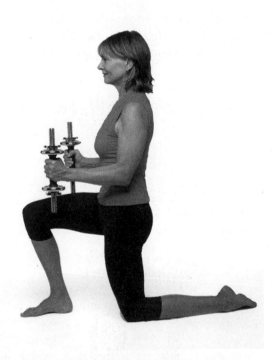

In starting position, connect with all your principles of alignment.

Anchors

Here are your anchor points:

-   Your shoulder girdle stabilization from positioning, with your shoulder blades locked onto your rib cage in back

- The foot of one leg and the knee of your other leg on the floor

- Your abdominals engaged and your pelvis anchored

Isolate

Keeping the 90-degree bend at your elbows, exhale to deeply activate your abdominals and raise your arms in front of you until your elbows are slightly lower and slightly wider than your shoulders.

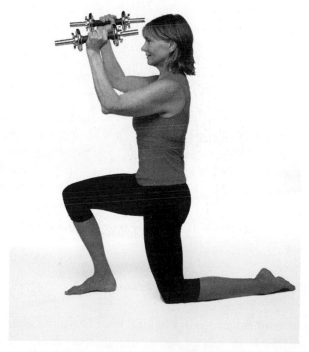

Raising your elbows with your shoulders anchored down immediately isolates the muscles of your shoulders that you're targeting with Fit Quickie #14.

Repetitions

Here's what to do:

1. With a light grasp on the weights in your hands, lift the weights 2 inches toward the ceiling and back down 2 inches for 12 to 15 repetitions in that small range of motion. Each 2-inch lift should take about 1 second, and each move back to the starting point should take 1 second.

2. After the last repetition, slowly lower your arms back to starting position.

3. Pause for 15 seconds and take a breath, rolling your shoulders to release any tension and reconnecting with your anchors.

4. Exhale and draw the weights back up to shoulder height. Inhale and lower them back to your sides, keeping the 90-degree bend at your elbow. Each lift should take about 2 seconds, and each lowering phase should take about 2 seconds. Complete 8 to 10 repetitions.

Rest for 15 seconds, change legs, and repeat from the start.

 Although you can do this exercise seated or standing, the kneeling position serves another purpose: it requires you to recruit more core muscles to maintain position as you find yourself slightly struggling for balance. This steps up the challenge to your abdominals, gluteals, and back muscles.

Stretch

Now for your stretch:

1. Lightly connect your fingertips low behind your back, and gently reach them down and back toward the floor behind you to stretch your shoulders.

2. If your hands don't meet, simply reach your arms in the direction of the floor behind you. Hold for 20 to 30 seconds.

Common Errors

Beware of these common errors while you exercise:

- Don't allow your shoulder blades to leave their anchor point on your back.

- Don't allow your shoulders to sneak up toward your ears as your upper trapezius muscle tries to help with the workload. If this happens, stop, drop your elbows back to their position at your side, roll your shoulders and reset their position, and resume the repetitions.

- Don't allow your pelvis to slip into an anterior tilt. Keep your abdominals braced and your gluteals engaged in support of your pelvic anchor.

Tips and Modifications

These tips and alternate ways to perform the exercise might help:

- To deepen the challenge to your abdominals and the other muscles of your core, place the foot of your front leg in a direct line forward of your knee on the floor. This is very destabilizing and will make your core muscles really scramble to help you keep your balance!

- When you can easily do the repetitions with the weights you're using, increase them by 1 pound in each hand as you work your way up, or increase your repetitions. Remember the 90-second rule from the earlier "The Exercise Prescription" chapter.

- Always start with low weights and low reps and work your way up. Begin without dumbbells as you work on your form. Then add 1-pound weights. When you can do 15 repetitions with 1-pound weights in each hand, progress to 2-pound weights, and so on. Be aware that, as the weight you lift increases, the number of repetitions you can practice in good form drops as you work your way up again. Remember, form always trumps reps.

As important as it is to strengthen the anterior muscles of your shoulders for good strength, shape, and function—as this exercise does—remember that your posterior shoulder muscles are just as hungry for your attention. Challenge should always be teamed with balance. If your exercise routine sidesteps the back of your shoulders in favor of working the front, it's time to even the score. Let Fit Quickie #14 claim an even number of places on your targeted muscles dance card.

WINDING UP YOUR WILLPOWER

Oh sure, you start the day motivated. You'll eat right and work out today! Then all of a sudden, it's noon and you succumb to that tray of pastries in the break room. Or you drive straight home after work to hit the couch, watching the gym fade rapidly in the rearview mirror, despite your best-laid plans to exercise today after work.

Willpower. Sometimes you have it; other times it's nowhere to be found. In stressful situations, dietary pledges and even the best-laid exercise plans can quickly disappear. For truly healthy living, you need to find ways to relieve stress and restore your emotional equilibrium.

As it turns out, willpower comes in limited supply. So although you might have the best intentions about eating healthy and exercising, stress hammers away at your willpower until you can feel like there isn't any left, report R. Baumeister and team in the *Journal of Personality and Social Psychology,* 2008. The traffic makes you late to work. You drop and shatter your favorite coffee mug. You have a fight with your coworker. You know you should say "no" to that cheesecake in the break room, but …. It goes on and on.

What you're experiencing is a struggle between your stress-relieving impulse to indulge in a "treat" and your willpower to abstain. It's not your fault. The impulse is driven by your momentary cravings—a stress-management tactic—that's recalling your previous experiences of how to turn a bad day into a mini pleasure cycle. And acts of self-control, or those that demand some degree of willpower, consume substantial quantities of glucose. This results in a drop in your blood sugar, which drives up your interest in food, confirm M. Gailliot and his research team in 2007 in *The Journal of Personality and Social Psychology.* No wonder you crave that candy bar!

Although your willpower reserve drains in the face of stress, it's a renewable resource and can be replenished with just 5 minutes of exercise or meditation.

Even if you caved on the candy bar, if you were even faintly aware that there was a bit of a struggle going on, that's good news. It shows you have something upon which to build a different ending. As a human, you are gifted with the self-awareness that allows you to make a choice—a choice for immediate gratification or a choice in your greater best interests, compatible with your big-picture, long-term goals of a healthier body and a trimmer waist. It's as if, according to K. Vohs and team, as reported in *Social and Personality Psychology Compass* in 2007, you have two selves with competing motivations. Neuroscientists refer to it as one brain but two minds. And one of them has to prevail.

In the midst of the struggle, it helps to realize that both of these urges—the impulsive self and self-control—have always been a part of your psyche. Your twenty-first-century brain still zeroes in on something fat and sweet-tasting because, in leaner times, the energy load these foods provide ensured survival.

At the same time, your self-control system has evolved in your brain's prefrontal cortex, reports R. Sapolsky in *Philosophical Transactions of the Royal Society of London* in 2004. This is the willpower tool that allows you to override immediate temptation with better judgment. You've implemented that tool successfully on multiple occasions, so you know it's there. The trick is figuring out how to have more willpower wins than instant-gratification indulgences so you can fit into that favorite pair of jeans, finish that project, or get in some exercise.

The Fit Quickie Fix

Failure to follow through on the best-laid plans can be disheartening. What happened to your dietary promise, your commitment to getting your workout done today, your pledge to clean out that closet or finish that least-favored project at work?

Fortunately, you don't have to just keep your fingers crossed and hope you'll do better next time. Specific strategies can make your willpower muscle mightier and help reinforce your best-interests instinct.

No wonder we call ourselves stress eaters. High-fat, high-sugar food produces a cascade of biological pleasure responses that quickly rescue you from the pain of stress. The great news is, there are proven ways you can strengthen your willpower and stop sabotaging yourself on the way to realizing your health, weight loss, and fitness goals.

According to Kelly McGonigal, PhD, author of *The Willpower Instinct*, both exercise and meditation restore the executive command center of your brain that manages impulse control.

So you thought Fit Quickies were all about body shaping? Guess again. They're also about *brain* shaping. A 5-minute Fit Quickie not only lifts your bum, but also sharpens your brainpower. Even better: *any* exercise will do it. The willpower-strengthening benefits of physical activity are immediate in reducing cravings and overall stress, enhancing self-control, and making your brain function faster. And exercise accomplishes all this by, among other things, enhancing the activity of your brain's prefrontal cortex—a.k.a., willpower central.

Physical activity not only changes your mood and reduces stress—which is the number-one enemy of self-control and willpower—but it also changes your brain in many of the same ways meditation does. It seems to literally build neural density in the areas of your brain that are important for self-control, improving blood flow in those regions and making them better connected and less easily fatigued. Getting your circulation going makes your brain stronger and better able to exert focus and self-control in a wide range of domains, whether it's resisting temptation or just paying attention.

The long-term effects of exercise are even more impressive: workouts enhance your biology of self-control by restoring variability to your heart rate. That's a fancy way of saying exercise delivers you from a chronic state of fight-or-flight stress that somehow manages to rev up your system into a chronic stress state, according to Kelly McGonigal in *The Willpower Instinct*.

How to Do It

When it comes to reconstructing willpower, your brain and body don't care what you do, as long as you do it. For flexing your prefrontal cortex, everything from doing energetic housekeeping, to making a mad dash to the departure gate, to taking the stairs instead of the elevator counts. Considering that barely 10 percent of Americans meet suggested standards for physical activity, it's no wonder stress and rampant overeating of junk food and other destructive yet compelling activities have become so problematic.

Exercising to Build Willpower

Boosting your willpower with exercise doesn't demand much time. In a 2010 report by J. Barton and J. Pretty in *Environmental Science and Technology* analyzing 10 different studies, it was demonstrated that the greatest mood-boosting and stress-reducing effects of exercise come from just 5-minute chunks of exercise. That's right—you don't need to invest in an hour-long workout to get the benefits. Sounds like a job for Fit Quickies!

Today, find at least 5 minutes to devote to an outdoor stroll, your favorite Fit Quickie, a few minutes of yoga, or your preferred method of exercise. You'll work your body, your brain, and your willpower.

Meditating to Build Willpower

Anxiety is a good catch-all term for mounting stress, uncertainty, and the wild array of uncontrollables we call life. I don't need to tell you how easy it is to get caught in the muddle. Your brain, it turns out, is especially vulnerable to temptation when you're feeling bad. When you're feeling down, what do you do to feel better? If you're like most people, you turn to the promise of reward.

Remember, mounting stress chips away at your willpower, leading to cravings and all kinds of other behaviors you know are the exact opposite of what's compatible with your weight-loss, health, and body-shaping goals. That's the bad news. The good news is that there is a way out.

With meditation, you become startlingly aware of how habituated your responses to stress are. You start to see, as you find yourself between urge and action, that you have a choice of what action you take. Even the simplest meditation practice increases your awareness of this moment and bolsters your ability to make better choices at critical moments.

According to the American Psychological Association, the most commonly used strategies for dealing with stress are those that activate your brain's reward system: eating, drinking, shopping, watching TV, surfing the web, and playing video games.

A simple meditation practice can directly reduce the effects of anxiety. It disentangles you from the mess and restores calm and perspective—which is a neurological response to the meditation process. And you don't have to "believe in" anything for it to work. You don't have to light a candle or create any special sacred place. If you can breathe, you're in.

You can utilize several simple techniques for meditation. I've taught a simple, restorative meditation in my fitness classes for years that recharges the executive command center of your brain in just 5 minutes:

1. Sit comfortably in a chair or on a floor cushion, or lie down—but don't fall asleep!

2. Close your eyes.

3. Let your bones drop into the chair or cushion. Remain alert yet relaxed.

4. Bring your attention to your breath at either your nose, belly, or throat. Every time you notice that your mind has wandered—and it will—without judgment, bring your attention back to focus on your breath. The more your mind wanders, the more you get to practice coming back. This process of concentration with the return of focus builds your willpower muscle.

5. Sit still, without moving. When the urge to shift positions hits, don't move. This trains you to find the pause between stimulus and habituated response, which is the exact point of making choices. By flexing this muscle during meditation, you strengthen it just like any other muscle. Practicing not scratching that itch or shifting on your cushion translates directly into not eating that cookie. You learn to acknowledge the urge without acting upon it.

Start with 5 minutes of meditation every day for a week. Just commit to that much. If your mind keeps wandering during your meditation, that's okay. It's all about the practice of returning to your point of concentration. If you miss a day, that's okay, too. Just pick up your practice the next day. Let go of that perfectionist anxiety just as you let go of wandering thoughts, and come back to your breath. This mindfulness restocks your willpower reserves.

Another powerful restorative choice is guided relaxation. With guided relaxation, you mentally walk through a body-relaxation process, limb by limb. Your focus of concentration as you move through your body is the key element. This, coupled with releasing tension, can be a real game-changer when it comes to stress management. You can do guided meditation on your own or follow along with an audio guide.

 For *Lani's Dessert,* a 12-minute guided relaxation audio program that restores mental and emotional equilibrium, go to lanimuelrath.com.

Developing a meditation practice (more about this in the later "Motivation and Mind-Set for Success" chapter) and getting the support of a coach were pivotal and essential factors in my 50-pound weight loss. Yes, exercise and diet are critical—they are the physical tools, and I absolutely couldn't have done it without them. But mind-set and meditation practice make a difference and might well be your missing link. Whether you practice my 5-step meditation, guided relaxation, or another technique, the effects will sneak up on you in surprising and delightful ways.

CREATING FIT QUICKIE ROUTINES

Are you fired up about Fit Quickies and ready to add them to your workouts? Of course you are! Let's look at how you can incorporate Fit Quickies into your day or your current workout rotations.

Incorporating muscle-challenging workouts into your day and benefiting from the increased strength, shape, and vitality they deliver is easier than you might think. I like short, focused workouts that really target certain muscles so I can work on my strength and shape and then get on with enjoying life in a well-challenged body. In fact, that's the foundation of the whole Fit Quickie philosophy: go deep and go home!

If you're a workout veteran, I'm betting you've already tried a few Fit Quickies and are well on your way to building your own list of favorites. They will add a fresh dimension to your current workouts. Mix them into what you're doing now, or switch them out on alternate resistance training days for something new.

I've created some sample Fit Quickie routines to help you get started. I've suggested some short combinations—Fit Quickie "bundles"—for those days when you can squeeze in only 10 minutes of exercise intermittently through the day, and to lend enthusiastic support for your antisedentary campaign. You'll discover a few combinations for targeting specific zones, such as the lower or upper body.

I've also created some routines you can do in "superset" fashion. Supersets are one of my favorite methods for getting a full-body strength-training workout in a short chunk of time—about 25 minutes, including stretches.

And if you're just starting to exercise, I have some suggestions for how you can get started, too.

10-Minute Fit Quickie Bundles

Let's start with some 10-minute combinations. So much flexibility and fun is built into the Fit Quickies that you'll soon get the knack of whipping up fun combinations on your own.

Each bundle takes about 10 minutes. Complete three or four bundles over the course of a day in 10-minute chunks, and by day's end, you can put a star on your to-do chart next to "resistance training workout" for the day. Remember, you're after resistance training that challenges your muscles two or three times a week, depending on your goals and condition. I encourage you toward three times per week.

Fit Quickie Bundle #1: Instant Invigorator

Fit Quickie #10: Legs into Play

Fit Quickie #4: Gorgeous Glutes and Hamstrings

Fit Quickie #11: Upper-Body SOS

Fit Quickie Bundle #2: Bums and Tums

Fit Quickie #1: 7 Seconds to a Flat Belly

Fit Quickie #5: Topless Muffins

Fit Quickie #8: Tush Tighteners

Fit Quickie Bundle #3: Full-Body Recharger

Fit Quickie #11: Upper-Body SOS

Fit Quickie #3: Triceps Triple Play

Fit Quickie #12: Super-Shaper Split Squats

Fit Quickie Bundle #4: Laser Lower Body

Fit Quickie #10: Legs into Play

Fit Quickie #6: Thigh Warriors

Fit Quickie #9: Higher Assets

These are a few examples, but the possibilities are endless. Just be sure you're warmed up at the beginning of the bundle, and you're good to go.

 You can almost use a pick-up-sticks approach to Fit Quickies bundle planning. Assemble 15 small paper cards. Write a Fit Quickie number on each of the cards. Divide the entire stack into two piles, one with all the upper-body-focused Fit Quickies, the other with the lower-body-focused sequences. Grab one or two from each pile, and you have a unique combination. Fit Quickies with an upper-body focus include #2, #3, #11, and #14. Fit Quickies with a lower-body focus include #4, #5, #6, #7, #8, and #9. Fit Quickies #1 and #7 have an abdominals focus. And don't forget Fit Quickie #11, which works those abdominals isometrically as stabilizers, too.

When building your own Fit Quickie bundles, remember to respect two important considerations:

Warm up your muscles first, for best performance. You can do this within the Fit Quickies themselves, and that's why I often start Fit Quickie bundles with Fit Quickie #10. It fires up all the muscles of your lower body and stimulates circulation through your entire body quite quickly. Lightly loaded push-ups can do the same for your upper body. Do a few standing push-ups against the wall to stimulate circulation in your upper extremities before doing more challenging push-ups or planks on the floor, or prior to Fit Quickie #14.

Your body-shaping benefit is in direct proportion to your effort at the end. At the end of your repetitions for each Fit Quickie, your muscles should feel maxed out. It should be difficult for you to manage another repetition or two in good form. Short, hard workouts can be your best body-shaping and time-saving friend. You just have to play by the rules. And depending on your individual condition, that muscle max will come at a different point and a different resistance load than it will for someone else.

Focused Fit Quickie Sequences

Another way to mix and match Fit Quickies is to group them according to target areas. This allows you to approach the same muscle groups in a way that challenges them from a variety of angles, making the workload more diverse and keeping things fun, too. Remember warm-ups and the all-important capital-E, *Effort*, by the end of the set.

Lower-Body Fit Quickie Sequence #1 (18 minutes):

> Fit Quickie #10: Legs into Play
>
> Fit Quickie #6: Thigh Warriors
>
> Fit Quickie #4: Gorgeous Glutes and Hamstrings
>
> Fit Quickie #5: Topless Muffins

Lower-Body Fit Quickie Sequence #2 (15 minutes):

> Fit Quickie #10: Legs into Play
>
> Fit Quickie #12: Super-Shaper Split Squats
>
> Fit Quickie #9: Higher Assets
>
> Fit Quickie #8: Tush Tighteners

Lower-Body Fit Quickie Sequence #3 (22 minutes):

> Fit Quickie #10: Legs into Play
>
> Fit Quickie #4: Gorgeous Glutes and Hamstrings
>
> Fit Quickie #9: Higher Assets
>
> Fit Quickie #5: Topless Muffins
>
> Fit Quickie #2: Inner Thigh Squeeze and Tease

Create your own Fit Quickie combinations, including your favorites, and be sure you also challenge yourself with those that aren't. Chances are, they're challenging you in the places you need it most.

The Full-Body Fit Quickie Workout

It's easy to build a Fit Quickie full-body workout that you can complete in 20, 30 or 45 minutes, depending on how many sets you do and how long you take for rest intervals between exercises. These all vary depending on your current condition.

Keep in mind that you're striving to get the most benefit from each set. You need enough recovery time between exercises that you have vitality for the next exercise, yet without so much rest that you lose the momentum of your workout session altogether.

Full-Body Fit Quickie Workout Routine #1 (38 minutes):

> Fit Quickie #1: 7 Seconds to a Flat Belly
>
> Fit Quickie #10: Legs into Play
>
> Fit Quickie #11: Upper-Body SOS
>
> Fit Quickie #3: Triceps Triple Play
>
> Fit Quickie #4: Gorgeous Glutes and Hamstrings
>
> Fit Quickie #5: Topless Muffins
>
> Fit Quickie #6: Thigh Warriors
>
> Fit Quickie #7: Kickstand Core Challenge
>
> Fit Quickie #13: Back Beauty
>
> Fit Quickie #8: Tush Tighteners

Full-Body Fit Quickie Workout Routine #2 (50 minutes):

Fit Quickie #10: Legs into Play

Fit Quickie #2: Inner Thigh Squeeze and Tease

Fit Quickie #3: Triceps Triple Play

Fit Quickie #4: Gorgeous Glutes and Hamstrings

Fit Quickie #5: Topless Muffins

Fit Quickie #6: Thigh Warriors

Fit Quickie #7: Kickstand Core Challenge

Fit Quickie #9: Higher Assets

Fit Quickie #11: Upper-Body SOS

Fit Quickie #12: Super-Shaper Split Squats

Fit Quickie #14: Shoulder Shapers

 When building your own full-body Fit Quickie workouts, make it a point to vary the order and alternate your lead leg. For example, in the audio and video downloads available at lanimuelrath.com, the instructions lead off with the same leg each time—such are the necessities of recordings. In practice, it's best to alternate leads, to keep the workload more varied and foster muscle balance.

Full-Body Fit Quickie Superset Routines

Supersets enable you to keep moving during resistance training, cutting your workout time by shortening the rest phase you need between sets. With supersets, you alternate muscle group challenges, allowing one set of muscles to recover while you target another area. For example, you might complete one Fit Quickie that focuses on your lower body and follow it with another Fit Quickie that targets your upper body. Then you can go back to your lower body for another set—or another lower-body sequence—while your upper-body muscles recover.

The important thing to remember is to pace yourself carefully enough that you approach no set exhausted, out of breath, or, worse yet, out of form. Control and precision are still vital to best results.

With supersets, exercises that alternate on your upper and lower body become chained together into a complete workout. You perform each team of exercises, called a sequence, one or two times before moving onto the next sequence. Again, it provides for a limitless variety of sequences as you mix and match exercises, keeping your body—and your brain— challenged, the must-haves when it comes to building strength and a beautiful shape.

Chunking the exercises in this fashion is also a psychological plus because you can mentally check off sections of the workout as "done!" while you go. With supersets, the time always goes fast, and you won't believe how many muscles you're able to challenge in such a short time, resurrecting your energy and restoring your physical confidence for the rest of your day ahead.

There are an infinite number of ways to combine Fit Quickies into supersets. Here are two of my favorite series, to give you an idea. After practicing these sequences a few times, you'll get the hang of alternating muscle groups and hopefully become inspired to mix and match your own combinations. Just remember, variety is key to keeping your muscles guessing!

Fit Quickie Superset Routine Series #1:

Time: 25 minutes, including stretches (The stretches all fall at the end of the series so you can keep moving.)

Warm-up: Fit Quickie #10; Fit Quickie #2, standing, 1 set

Sequence 1:

1. Upper body: Fit Quickie #11: push-ups, either on knees or with straight legs, as many as you can do with strict form.

2. Lower body: Fit Quickie #12, 12 reps each leg.

3. Repeat steps 1 and 2.

Sequence 2:

1. Upper body: Fit Quickie #13.

2. Exercise D: (lower body): Fit Quickie #4.

3. Fit Quickie #5.

Sequence 3:

1. Fit Quickie #11, planks: rest 15 seconds, repeat.

2. Fit Quickie #8.

Stretches:

1. Upper-back stretch from Fit Quickie #13.

2. Hip and back stretch from Fit Quickie #4.

3. Half-lotus and waist stretch from Fit Quickie #5.

4. Pectoral stretch from Fit Quickie #11.

5. Hamstring stretch from Fit Quickie #8.

Fit Quickie Superset Routine Series #2:

Time: 25 minutes, including stretches (The stretches all fall at the end of this series so you can keep moving.)

Warm-up: Fit Quickie #10

Sequence 1:

1. Lower body: Fit Quickie #12, 12 reps each leg.

2. Upper body: Fit Quickie #14.

3. Repeat steps 1 and 2.

Sequence 2:

1. Lower body: Fit Quickie #9.

2. Upper body: Fit Quickie #3.

3. Repeat steps 1 and 2.

Sequence 3:

1. Fit Quickie #7.

2. Fit Quickie #8.

Increasing the Intensity of Fit Quickies

In each Fit Quickie, you position your body in a specific posture and work with precision. Always remember PAIR—position, anchor, isolation, and repetitions—as you work. These specifics invite maximum muscle effort, and being vigilant about maintaining these details is an important component of the challenge.

 When it comes to building strength and shape, evidence suggests it's the effort in the muscle produced at the *end* of the set that counts. This intensity of effort is largely a function of proper position—and focus!

Your body will quickly want to let go of alignment to ease the workload. This urge to kick back shows up in various ways: a leg moving out of the work zone by sneaking out of alignment into release, or your shoulder blades sliding forward off your back during push-ups as your upper-back stabilizers get tired and want to check out of the project. Vigilance!

Paying attention to these details keeps your muscle challenge sufficient for an indefinite period of time. After that, your options to increase your challenge include boosting the amount of resistance in a variety of ways. With Fit Quickies that utilize hand weights, you can gradually increase the weight you use. With Fit Quickies relying on body weight for resistance, such as push-ups or planks, you can increase the resistance by going to a more advanced version of the basic position. Several Fit Quickies, such as Fit Quickie #4, also lend themselves to additional resistance via the use of ankle weights. Get creative, think form above all else, and be precise.

If You're New to Exercise

If you're returning from a long workout "vacation" or are just getting started with resistance training, Fit Quickies are a perfect starting place. I've already broken them into bite-size chunks. I don't want you to wait another minute before enjoying all the body and mind benefits that moving your body against resistance can deliver.

Before you do anything, though, check with your health-care provider to be sure you're cleared to start resistance exercise. Then begin with Fit Quickie #1—either sitting, lying, or standing—and start building a connection to your core muscles. You'll also enjoy the added advantage of entering into a simple, deep-breathing pattern that will pay off immediately in stress protection, restored well-being, and increased willpower for moving forward with healthy plans.

You can practice Fit Quickie #1 every day—it takes only about 3 minutes! When you have the hang of that, pick another Fit Quickie that looks doable to you. Study the instructions and begin to practice it every other day. When you've got these two exercises under your belt, pick a third. Soon you'll be mixing and matching Fit Quickies like a pro.

Let it be a time for a new approach, a new perspective. Have fun, and always keep your sense of humor.

NUTRITION PRINCIPLES

If you can get control of your diet, you can get control over more than you ever imagined possible. Think about it. If you say you want to "get healthy" or "lose weight," what you're really looking for is control over your physical confidence, your energy, your protection from disease, and your figure, right? You're raising your hand and saying that you want the freedom and independence that, bottom line, depend on your health and weight. And more than any other single factor, your health and weight depend on what you put on your fork.

Research overwhelmingly supports a whole-food, plant-based, low-fat diet as the superior option for achieving optimum health and weight. Every day, I receive questions from people who want to know how to get started eating a plant-based diet for weight loss and fitness. In this chapter, I share the secrets of this wonderful way of eating—and living—with you.

A Foundation of Healthy Living

Perhaps the best way to tell you about plant-based eating is to tell you about my own journey. Actually, this is the focus of this chapter—to give you the benefit of my experience—not from the perspective of a dietitian, but as someone who sought and struggled for years to find the solution to a weight problem that was compatible with my highest ideals. Hopefully, my story can help you bypass some of the detours I had to endure. I share some important insights into why this food plan works for healthy and easy weight management, critical lessons from the experts and the research, and tips for speeding things up so you can get slim without all the roadblocks.

For starters, let's look at what a whole-foods, plant-based, low-fat diet really is.

Whole foods are unprocessed, or minimally processed, before they're consumed. They do not contain added ingredients such as salt, sugars, or fat. An example of a whole food is an orange. In contrast, orange juice is refined and processed and no longer "whole" because the juice of the orange is separated and extracted from the fiber. An example of minimally processed food is a whole oat coarsely chopped into oat groats, or whole grains coarsely ground into coarse flour, retaining their fiber.

A *plant-based diet* is one in which the majority (if not all) of your dietary energy, or calories, are derived from plant foods. This includes vegetables, starchy vegetables, grains, fruits, beans and legumes, and nuts and seeds.

A *low-fat diet* is largely centered on whole plant foods because the majority of whole plant foods are low in fat. However, there are some exceptions. Some plant foods—avocados, olives, nuts, and seeds—are quite high in fat. They pack a lot of energy into a small space, and if weight loss is your goal, you should consume these foods in moderation. My whole-food, plant-based diet eliminates many edibles that are high in fat—dairy products, meat, fish, eggs, and oils (which are 100 percent fat).

 Vegetable oils are extremely low in nutritive value. A processed food expelled from fibrous vegetables, fruits, and nuts, these oils contain 120 calories per tablespoon and easily contribute to overconsumption of calories.

My Journey

My diet history is littered with dog-eared diet books, stacks of journals, and plenty of excess pounds, not to mention lots of tears and incessant hunger.

Fifteen years ago, I weighed my most—190 pounds. Today I weigh 50 pounds less than I did then. Getting to where I am now has been a journey perhaps not unlike your own.

I have a genetic predisposition toward easy weight gain. I'm slow to lose weight, and I love to eat. So when it comes to easy weight management, the details of what I eat matter more than they might for someone who has never been weight challenged. My success hangs in the balance between energy intake and satisfaction from what I eat. The question is, how do you eat so you can be healthy, full, but not fat?

The exciting thing is that there's a simple, delicious way to eat that provides this solution. This way of eating also addresses health, and the natural outcome of a healthy, optimal diet is a healthy weight. All the uncertainties are taken out of it when you eat whole, plant foods.

To get things off to a reassuring start, here's a quote from one of the interviews I conducted while preparing this book. I think it's worth framing for your kitchen:

> I tell people there's your starchy vegetables, whole grains, and legumes as your foundation. Pick from any of those based on your preference, and then add lots of vegetables and some fruits. If you can do that for the rest of your life and make that where most, if not all, of your calories come from, then you're going to do really, really well. So it's just about trying to keep it very simple.
>
> —Matthew Lederman, MD

Don't you just love the simplicity in this? And if you ever get too caught up worrying about the food on your plate, return to this quote and take comfort. With these words as your foundation, the doors to eating freedom and enjoying a trim body are wide open.

Now for those personal details I promised: I've been eating a vegetarian diet for nearly 40 years. What I eat within the vegetarian realm has shifted, however, and that has played an important role in my weight-loss success. Over the years, despite multiple attempts and a variety of vegetarian eating plans for losing weight that gave me only intermittent success, I kept trying.

Through all those years of hit-and-miss, two underlying convictions prevailed:

My hunger signals couldn't be wrong or faulty. I figured something must be wrong with the *system*—not my body—if I needed to weigh or measure everything. Something's wrong with the system if I have to addle my brain with counting 1.73 grams protein and 2.426 grams carbohydrates, or any other living-your-life-as-a-lab system. Yet without a guiding set of principles to navigate the challenges, and given the dizzying array of dietary plans, my weight problem persisted.

There must be a way to eat that would allow me to use hunger and fullness signals as my guide. The squirrels and deer grazing in the mountains where I live don't count or measure anything. They don't have to use external tricks or devices to get themselves into some kind of zone. And they don't have to try to figure out how to eat less. They have plenty to eat, and most times they aren't fat.

What had they figured out, without really thinking about it, that I hadn't? Sure, I knew about calories. Most of the diets I'd tried over the years had some sort of calorie-counting component, and I could manage my weight with portions and counting … for a while. But it was hard, and I was hungry.

Yet even with this conviction, my diet—depending on where I was with my success at micromanaging calories via one method or another—kept me intermittently padded with excess weight. What was I missing?

A Major Turn of Events

My search finally brought me to an eating coach who helped me take a big leap forward. By this point, years of frustration had me wanting, more than anything, to have a healthy, happy relationship with food, eating, and my body. What appealed to me about the work of Jean Antonello, obesity and eating disorder specialist, was that the central theme to her approach dovetailed with my hopes about hunger, fullness, and appetite. The focus of Jean's program, *Naturally Thin*, is how to stop dieting and become naturally thin by cooperating with your body: tuning in to your body's hunger signals, eating quality food every time you get hungry, and stopping when your body says "Stop." You can see why this appealed to me because it never seemed right to me that I would have a weight problem if I satisfied my hunger. Why would my body be designed so I had to connive and manipulate just to be a normal weight?

 Before making any substantial changes to your diet, especially if you're ill or are currently taking any medications, consult your health-care provider.

I wholeheartedly got onboard. The only rules I established, besides my vegetarian guidelines, were the basics from my coach:

- Eat every time I got hungry.

- Eat until I was full of quality, real food.

It made sense, it satisfied hunger, and it broke me from the enervating cycle of dieting. Eating this way both was a relief and produced a great deal of anxiety. Letting go of many of my previous restraints around food was scary. At first, I gained weight—a lot of weight— 40 pounds. As you can imagine, this wasn't without its challenges. As a college professor, fitness trainer, and physical educator, I was in front of people all the time, teaching exercise classes and lecturing. One aerobics student even asked me if I was pregnant. Yikes.

What kept me going? Intuitively, I knew I was on the right track.

Redefining "Quality" Food

Yet knowing what I know now, all that weight gain with getting off cycles of dieting would not have been necessary if I had been eating according to the dietary guidelines I now embrace.

The difference is that now I have a different view of what "high-quality" food means to me. At the time, I was eating a vegetarian diet and minimizing processed foods. Although refined, processed foods weren't considered "quality" according to my guidelines, dairy products, eggs, and vegetable oils were. "Moderate" fat intake, at about 20 percent of daily calories, was advised. Still, I gained weight. I was eating according to hunger and fullness signals, and my coach said that even though I would gain initially, eventually my weight would plateau and then slowly start to drop. This actually did happen, to some extent, because of the overall improvement in the quality of food I was eating and the fact that I wasn't undereating and overeating. But I was still missing some critical pieces of the puzzle.

Before going on, I want to underscore that I am deeply grateful to Jean because she taught me a lot about listening to my body and understanding that my body is not my enemy. The truth is, something is wrong with the food and the eating, not with my body. The fact that my body stored fat more readily than someone else's is not a design flaw; it's a genetic survival plus. I "got a good one," she'd say. This experience was an important step in helping me realize my goal: being well fed, slim, and healthy, with a healthy, happy relationship with food, eating, and my body. It drove home forever for me that the formula for success is about more than just the food. It's also about eating behaviors—eating enough and eating on time. Integrating these principles with my own dietary approach has been critical in helping me find my way.

Even after losing a bit of weight by eating according to hunger and fullness, I was still heavier than I wanted to be. So I began to implement some adjustments that would assist with weight loss. I lowered my calorie intake by eating smaller portions, yet I was careful not to cut them too dramatically. I knew too well the consequences of doing so—I would become hungry and restart the terrible ordeal of hunger management.

I was able to nudge my weight down a bit more, yet without the serious dietary controls or rebound hunger I experienced before. Still, I had faith that I would eventually find the solution that meant I wouldn't have to count anything.

Before this change of events, I had pored over books featuring a low-fat, vegetarian approach to health and weight management, including *The McDougall Plan*, by John McDougall, MD. Dr. McDougall is a pioneer in eating a whole-foods, plant-based, low-fat diet for health and weight loss. His plan appealed to my "eat when hungry until you're not" vision, and I eagerly jumped in. I lasted a few days, got hungry, and abandoned it.

I tried the high-volume/low-fat approach again a few years later, drawn by the sense and promise of it—eat according to appetite and be your natural thin weight—and again only lasted a few days.

To be fair, in retrospect, all the information I needed about what to eat was there. I just didn't see it. Plus, I needed help with the *how*. Sometimes it takes a village.

Breakthroughs in Eating Enlightenment

What finally made it all come together for me was a physician's seminar. This experience was a catalyst for me. I was able to take lessons I'd previously heard but not necessarily *learned*, implement appropriate action, and bring their health-building and pounds-off promise to life.

I was invited to attend an all-day nutrition conference. Dr. John McDougall took the stage for the entire afternoon, presenting documentation, graphs, slides, images, you name it to a roomful of cardiologists. His patience, clarity, and ability to make everything seem so commonsense had a disarming effect on the cardiologist crowd. And for me, it drove home points I'd heard before, yet I realized I hadn't quite gotten the full impact until that day. For example, I left that seminar with a deeper understanding of how vegetable oils and dairy products were no doubt standing in the way of my progress due to their high energy density. (More on energy density in a minute.)

Some of the greatest moments of enlightenment had to do with the importance of what I now affectionately call "starchies." I realized that, as much as I was *intellectually* convinced about the wisdom of the whole-foods, plant-based, low-fat plan and what a good match it was for my goals, my less-than-optimal history of results stemmed from me holding back on and not eating enough of the comfort foods—potatoes, yams, brown rice, and all their friends—in a way that was sabotaging my success. Although I professed to have given up carbophobia long before, apparently some residual influence was still hampering my progress.

Carbophobia, according to S. N. Cheuvront, PhD, RD, in a 2003 *Journal of the American of Nutrition* review of low-carb diets and theories, is "a form of nutrition misinformation infused into the American psyche through multiple advertising avenues that include magazine ads, television infomercials and especially best-selling diet books."

Full Without Being Fat

We long for hunger satisfaction—satiation—in a way that also keeps us naturally slim. Isn't that something we all want? The dieter's holy grail. Just the word *satiation* brings a sense of satisfaction and calm, doesn't it?

But what delivers satiation in a meal? And how can we get it so that we can eat to satisfaction and still stay slender? Isn't it necessary to stay a little hungry to drop some pounds? If your hunger is satisfied, you'll just retain your excess weight—or, even worse, gain weight—right? That's how it's been in the past. Better stick to your portions and tide yourself over on foods from the "unlimited" list.

Hunger and fullness need to be headlined in this conversation—that's been key for me. You may have heard that a whole-foods, plant-based diet keeps you slim, but you may not know why. I couldn't write this chapter without bringing this front and center. Understanding the why will make it easier for you to implement. Your focus will be clearer. It certainly made it so for me.

Satiation is satisfaction of appetite that results in the end of eating a meal. *Satiety* is the feeling of fullness that persists after eating, suppressing further consumption.

Multiple factors influence hunger satisfaction, many of which we understand and many of which we know little, if anything, about. Yet if you want to be full without being fat, you need to go three for three with what you put on your fork:

- Stretch

- Weight

- Energy

Let's look at stretch first. We know that gastric distension is an important element in hunger satisfaction. When you eat, the food in your gut stimulates nerves in your gastrointestinal tissues, called stretch receptors, firing off messages to your brain indicating that you've had enough to eat, as reported in 1982 by K. A. Houpt in the *Neuroscience Behavioral Review*.

Yet we also know that stretch alone doesn't do the trick. It's why a cabbage-and-cardboard diet doesn't work. You may get plenty of stretch, but if you've tried similar shenanigans to drop pounds, you know something's missing when it comes to hunger satisfaction.

So if it's not just the stretch factor, what else comes into play with hunger satisfaction? What else do you need to consider when seeking satiation when you eat, while still staying trim? In a word: weight. This one's a biggie. Research tells us that we tend to eat the same amount of weight in food every day, as reported by E. Bell and associates in 1998 in the *American Journal of Clinical Nutrition*. If you took everything you were to eat on any given day, tossed it into a basket, and weighed it, it would weigh the same as yesterday's basket, and tomorrow's basket, and the day after tomorrow's basket. Aha! Stretch and weight!

But here's the kicker: the weight-in-the-basket phenomenon can easily take precedence over how many calories the food in the basket contains. The implications here are enormous.

Time for a quick lesson on energy density: energy density is the energy content, or concentration of calories, per a given weight of food. For example, compare the calories in 1 pound of apples to 1 pound of chocolate or 1 pound of cheese.

Although they may take up about the same amount of space on a plate, I don't have to tell you that chocolate and cheese have a greater concentration of calories—higher *energy density* —pound for pound than the apples. If your goal is to fill up without getting fat, given a choice between the apples and the chocolates, which option is possibly going to allow you to surpass your calorie needs before you hit that standard of weight in your basket? Which is going to be more conducive to inviting your body to store excess body fat? They each deliver 1 pound of weight—but at significantly different calorie counts.

To take this further, which is going to give you better bang for your buck in the stretch receptor department? The chocolate will take up a lot less space when it hits your stomach because it's fiber free, for the most part, especially compared to the apples. Maybe you've never eaten a pound of apples in any one day, let alone at one sitting. As for chocolate, pounding down a mere 16 ounces of M&M's while casually running errands was nothing for me. Who do you think you're talking to?

A high-fat, energy-dense meal is usually much smaller in weight than a high-carbohydrate meal. So if you eat a constant amount of food, the high energy density of fat could be a key factor in overconsumption, report E. Bell and team at Pennsylvania State University, 1998.

Obviously, the apples trump the chocolate and the cheese when it comes to getting full without adding to your fat problem. Yet there's a breaking point. You've got stretch, and you've got weight. But guess what? There's another player in the satiety game.

Energy in the form of nutrient content gets a vote, too, according to J. A. Deutsch in a 1985 report in *The American Journal of Clinical Nutrition*. That means the calories in what you eat, for one thing. And I'm talking specifically about *enough* calories. Sometimes in our zealousness to cut calories, we forget how important it is to emphasize that the body needs sufficient amounts to function. It doesn't take any research data to tell me that if I cut calories too much, before long, it's going to catch up with me in the form of a bottomless, roaring appetite. Experience has taught me that one.

As it turns out, all three—stretch, weight, and energy—played a role in my years of falling short and my eventual success at being full without being fat. Yes, I was getting sufficient dietary fiber much of the time to trigger my stomach's stretch receptors—a critical part of the "feel full" picture. But I didn't pay sufficient attention to the food weight factor. Worse yet, before working with my coach, I repeatedly paid the price for undercutting calories, frequently offset by days of way too many calories without the benefit of the stretch and the food weight. I'd have, for example, 3 days of fruit and salads punctuated by a bowlful of cookie dough on Day 4. Perhaps you know the feeling.

Career dieters often have a knee-jerk negative response to the word *calories* because we've had such an antagonistic relationship with them in our quest to finding our ideal weight. But it's time to take a fresh look at calories for what they are, examine them in a new light, and see how they can actually be your friend. It's time to think differently because, as you now know, *calories don't stand alone* when it comes to finding the solution to your weight problem. If you become overenthused about cutting calories by eating only low-calorie food, you can have lots of fiber in your stomach but lack the calories you need to satisfy your hunger. Low fat can't work alone when it comes to weight loss. The persistent hunger that drove me to abandon my earlier attempts at whole-food, low-fat eating occurred because I wasn't honoring all the factors necessary to realize my goal of being able to lose weight while feeling well fed.

A similar problem occurs when consuming food high in calories, or energy density, that doesn't take up much space or weight—the chocolates instead of the apples. I don't know about you, but I've had my share of chocolate-instead-of-apples days.

 Apples and other fresh fruits weigh in at about 300 calories per pound, according to Lisle and Goldhammer in *The Pleasure Trap*. Compare that to the energy density of chocolate and cheese, at about 2,000 calories per pound, give or take.

This brings us to the heart of the whole-food, low-fat, plant-based food plan. We are biologically driven to satisfy our urge for a full belly because our bellies were designed to be satisfied with real, whole food. If you eat a lot of calorie-concentrated food—food high in energy density—that doesn't have much or any fiber, you can eat too many calories long before your hunger is satisfied, via the gastric stretch and food weight factors. Your hunger isn't the problem here; how you meet your hunger is. Because the weight factor of the food you eat is such a big part of satiation, you'll never reach your goals if you think you'll be satisfied according to hunger and fullness signals and you're counting on highly calorie-concentrated, processed foods to do it, according to K. Duncan and associates in a 1983 report in *The American Journal of Clinical Nutrition*.

 Although the stretch receptor phenomenon is one of the most obvious signs of fullness, activation of intestinal nutrient receptors are believed to play a role in satiety as well, say N. Read and team, in a 1994 *Nutrition Review* article.

Food weight, stomach stretch, and sufficient calorie intake are critical to your weight management success. Once you make friends with these key factors, you'll have a simple pathway to being healthy and lean for life. You'll be fully satisfied by what's on your plate easily, painlessly, and healthfully. All three pieces work together to give you satiation, or that "I've had enough" feeling. And more than that, they give you lasting satiety that carries you forward through your day. You need them all to be able to eat according to appetite and still be slim.

In contrast, high-caloric, low-volume foods without much bulk—or foods that don't take up much space in your digestive tract—whether concentrated in calories from their fat content or due to processing and elimination of fiber or water, present specific challenges when it comes to weight loss. You will easily overshoot your calorie needs long before you get the "I'm full!" feeling, according to Bell and team.

Do you see how this explains why you can cram down bags of potato chips without feeling the fullness you'd experience by eating the real deal, the whole potato? You just keep going until you reach a point at which you feel full—or beyond. And this comes at tremendous cost to your waistline.

And high-fat foods aren't the only problem. Foods highly concentrated in calories, like those fat-free yet highly processed and crammed-with-sugar cakes masquerading as muffins, are troublemakers, too. They pack enough calorie dynamite to blow your best body-shaping efforts clear out of the water.

 Bottom line: foods that squeeze a lot of calories into a tiny package have the potential to add lots of calories to your meal before you've had your fill.

Looking back, the biggest mistake I made in all those years of trying to lose weight was looking at calories without understanding the calorie companions in weight management, the stretch and the food weight factors. And not fully honoring my hunger signals.

From now on, I want you to think of these as four equal partners. When you do, it will revolutionize your relationship with food, eating, and your body. And it will lead you to your ideal weight with such steady certainty and joy, you'll wonder why you didn't team up this quartet—stretch, weight, energy, and honoring hunger signals—before.

Brilliant Success

The secret is to be discriminatory in your energy intake in a way that doesn't also drive up your hunger, backfiring in a binge. Promise me you'll kiss off those days of gritting your teeth through hunger signals or swearing allegiance to a rabbit-food diet, just to take off a paltry pound or two. No way. As a matter of fact, not consuming enough calories guarantees that you won't get where you want to be because you're so focused on keeping your calorie intake down. It's why eating only celery won't work. It's why counting calories or points alone won't work. When you've eating your caloric or "point" allotment in cookies, although you've met your calorie limit, you haven't met your fullness limit. So you keep eating.

Sticking with very low-calorie foods may be the rapid and logical conclusion to how to lose weight, but now you see why it's not the complete answer. The conditions of satiety have their stake in the game, too, and they tolerate no disrespect. You won't get enough calories to satisfy your hunger if you just eat fruits and vegetables. You can't hack your way into fat loss. If you've ever been on a white-knuckle hunger diet as I have, you know exactly what I mean. My experience at the physician's seminar brought this lesson into clear focus, and I knew what I had to do.

At my very next meal after leaving that seminar, I piled on the brown rice and potatoes with my vegetables, creating a perfect balance of stretch, weight, and calorie needs met. This is the magic of the whole-food, plant-based diet—still abundant in the high water content and color of the more perishable vegetables, yet sufficient in the more energy-dense starches.

I saw how calorie concentrated but fiber-free foods such as oils and dairy were causing me problems. That goes for other animal products, too, which are also often high in fat. These foods easily overshoot your calorie needs without giving you satiation. For me, consuming higher-quality foods meant I needed to be more prudent with the fats and fiber-free foods in my diet than I had been before.

The only "measuring" I did was to fill half of my dinner plate with rice, potatoes, or any other of a long list of starches and then fill the other half with steamed or stir-fried (easy and yummy without oil) vegetables using the eyeball method. This allowed me to eat according to my appetite, shed pounds, and get off the diet ride for good while eating mountains of delicious, whole, low-fat food. My rules of eating, as had been my ideal, now allowed me to stay slim: eat when hungry until you're not.

My Big-Plate Trick for Staying Trim

People ask me how to eat to lose weight. I never tell them exactly what to eat, yet I'm always happy to tell them exactly what and how *I* eat. Usually they ask me more than once because I don't think they quite believe that the solution is so simple.

I look at it this way: by day's end, if I were to take all the food I ate that day and put it on a big tray, half of it would be starchy veggies and whole grains, and the other half would be high-water-content vegetables. There would be about 1 cup or more beans, a few pieces of fruit on top, and a sprinkling of seeds. That's a good summation of my food each day, give or take. Over the course of weeks, some festive feast meals and treats would be thrown in, too. How much of that you can do depends on you and your weight-loss goals. It's not a religion, it's a guiding set of simple principles.

Meal by meal, it looks pretty much like this:

- Breakfast is usually whole grains and fruits.

- Lunch is a big bowl of soup with starchy vegetables, legumes, and dark greens or a salad—or both—often with a big sandwich on whole-grain bread.

- Dinner is a mountain of rice, potatoes, or another starchy vegetable, or pasta with another big pile of stir-fried or steamed veggies, and a salad.

 Forget the small plate rule. I call it my big plate trick for staying trim.

Somewhere during the day, I'll have more fruit. If I'm hungrier some days, I don't think twice about eating another plate of potatoes or grabbing a chunk of good grainy bread or more fruit. These foods aren't what makes you fat. But until you really understand about being well fed on these foods, you'll struggle with your hunger and, quite likely, your weight.

The Five Food Groups

My plant-based diet is organized around five food groups:

- Veggies

- Starchies

- Fruit

- Beans

- Nuts and seeds

The guiding principles are whole, low-fat, plant-based foods.

Following a whole-food, plant-based diet automatically gives you perfect amounts of protein, carbs, and fat. As long as you consume a variety of foods, you don't need to worry about calculating, weighing, measuring, or counting.
—Julieanna Hever, RD, *The Complete Idiot's Guide to Plant-Based Nutrition*

When it comes to veggies, opt for green and yellow, high-water-content vegetables. These are the ones you recognize as more perishable: leafy greens, cruciferous vegetables such as cabbage, broccoli, and cauliflower, and crispy colorfuls such as green and red peppers, onions, celery, and summer squash.

Starchies include starchy vegetables and whole grains. Sweet potatoes, yams, potatoes, corn, peas, winter squash, rice, oats, quinoa, pasta—the list is deliciously endless.

Fruit of all kinds—apples, oranges, plums, peaches, blueberries, raspberries, mango, pineapple, grapefruit, papaya, melon, grapes, cherries, and kiwi, for starters.

In the beans and legumes group, you'll find beans, lentils, and dried peas. Officially, these are starches, but because they have a higher protein content than starchy vegetables, I view them somewhat differently.

It's easy to get more protein than you need, especially if you eat animal products. Excess protein taxes your body, placing stress on your internal organs. Your body can't store protein like it can carbs or fat. About 1 cup a day from the beans and legumes group is a good amount to aim for so you get all the advantages of nutrition and satiety (although I don't measure, and if I eat more or less, that's just fine). Remember, there's protein in the vegetables, starches, and whole grains, too.

For nuts and seeds, aim for $\frac{1}{2}$ to 1 ounce a day, depending on your weight-loss and health goals. These foods can slow you down if you're trying to lose weight. Although they're a whole plant food, they're concentrated in calories and can contribute to weight gain.

A Typical Day's Menu

How does this all play out on the plate? How do you build it from the first meal of the day? Here's what my day looks like:

Breakfast: Usually, this is a large bowl of whole-grain cereal with berries, a banana, peaches, or some other juicy fruit on top. Sometimes it's pancakes or waffles, starchy vegetables, or a breakfast burrito.

Lunch: Generally, I eat a large bowl of soup with vegetables, starchies, and beans. In warmer weather, I opt for salad—either leafy greens or grated vegetables such as carrots and cabbage—instead of soup. Sometimes I have a veggie sandwich with hummus, tomato, or other vegetables on whole-grain bread. Or sometimes I have a salad *and* soup, depending on my appetite and how robust the soup is. Remember, your appetite can be your guide.

Dinner: This is usually a plate of half starchies and half veggies. It could be a heap of brown rice topped with steamed or stir-fried (without oil) vegetables, or a mountain of sweet potatoes or Yukon golds with a vegetable stir-fry. Again, I eyeball the portions and have more starchies if I'm so inclined.

All the ingredients are usually simple fare, which suits me just fine. I've also got an arsenal of yummy sauce and topping recipes to use when in the mood. I make veggie wraps, burritos, sweet potato lasagna, smoky butternut soup, and strawberry shortcake. This diversity and freedom is key. And the beauty of the way I eat is that I get all my essential nutrients (with the addition of vitamin B_{12}) without counting, weighing, or measuring. My goal is to eat according to my appetite and stay slim without obsessing and calculating every gram of macronutrient. Can it really be this simple? Yes.

In contrast to most vitamins, which are synthesized by plants, vitamin B_{12} is synthesized by bacteria growing in the soil, intestinal tracts of animals, and water. In our sanitized food environment, this bacteria has been cleaned from our plant food supply. According to Neal Barnard, MD, in the *21-Day Weight Loss Kickstart,* just 2.4 micrograms per day vitamin B_{12} is required for healthy adults. That's easy to get with a supplement or fortified foods.

If you're used to counting, weighing, and measuring and you find it too uncomfortable to let go of these controls all at once, that's understandable. At first, it can be frightening to think of what would happen if you let your body do the measuring. Think of it as a shift to *body-managed eating* (my coach called it *body-controlled eating*), turning over the control of how much and when to eat to your body. If you feel that simplifying to the five food groups is enough to help you get started and you'll tackle the "body managed" part later, that's no problem.

You can confidently turn over the management of when and how often to your body and stay slim when eating a whole-food, low-fat, plant-based diet. High-quality food is the key, though. You can't substitute a standard American diet (SAD). Processed, high-fat, fiber-deficient foods won't deliver satiation and satiety in a way that will keep you trim.

The Five Food Groups on My Plate

Here's how my five food group plan might play out over the course of a day. Keep in mind I don't weigh or measure my food, nor do I follow a prescribed diet of "portions," and I'm not telling you to, either. Yet to create a mental picture for you I think might be helpful, I've approximated a typical day with the following:

Veggies: 8 to 10+ servings, with 1 serving being 1 cup raw, leafy veggies or $\frac{1}{2}$ cup steamed/stir-fried veggies. With veggies in a salad or soup for lunch and more salad and steamed veggies for dinner, plus noshing on raw veggies as I prepare meals, I easily get 10+ servings a day.

Starchies: 8 to 10+ servings, with 1 serving being $\frac{1}{2}$ cup cooked whole grains or 1 small potato. By the time I've had $1\frac{1}{2}$ cups oatmeal for breakfast, potatoes or squash as a base for my soup at lunch, a sandwich, and a pile of brown rice or some type of potato with vegetables for dinner, I'm easily in for 8 to 10+ servings for the day.

Fruit: 3 or 4 servings, with 1 on my morning grains and more at various points during the day or perhaps as dessert.

Beans and legumes: 2+ servings, with 1 serving being $\frac{1}{2}$ cup cooked. Sometimes it's a little more, sometimes it's little less—remember, I'm not measuring. I'm approximating to give you a better idea of how it all works. I might have some beans in soup at lunch or with grains at dinner, sometimes mashed into a burger or as a spread via hummus, the new mayo, I get my 2+ servings.

Nuts and seeds: Up to 1 ounce a day. I often include about 1 tablespoon ground flaxseeds on my morning cereal. Sometimes I add walnuts, or for a richer dressing for vegetables, tahini.

What about condiments? I call these "decorations" because they're just that. The more your taste becomes realigned to whole, natural foods, the less you need the decorations. I enjoy my own flavor enhancers just like anyone else: a light sauce on my rice and veggies, dressing on salads, mustard on sandwiches, maple syrup on hotcakes, and ketchup on veggie burgers. It's what we do 90 percent of the time that matters, and that little wiggle room for fun can make a difference in creativity and how much you enjoy your meals.

One-Day Food Journal

Now let's look at exactly what I might eat during a day. This is a pretty typical day for me. Sometimes I eat these amounts; sometimes I eat more or less. I let my body tell me how much and how often.

Even though I used to be compelled to do same to manage my food plan, one of the big— I mean *big*—plusses of going whole foods, plant based, low-fat was no longer having to weigh or measure ever again and *still* stay trim and in good health.

But to give you an idea of how much I eat, I have measured here to encourage you with how much I do eat and to offset any ideas of limitation you might have. I also analyzed some totals of servings at the end, to compare them to my five food groups plan. I chose a day that was easy to quantify because it involved simple preparations. (Many days I have veggie wraps, hearty soups, pasta and sauce, or pancakes. These are harder to measure and report on, but it's just the same ingredients in fancier form.)

Breakfast:

> $1\frac{1}{2}$ cups cooked steel-cut oats
>
> $\frac{3}{4}$ cup blueberries
>
> 2 teaspoons ground flaxseeds

Lunch:

> 2 cups veggie stir-fry with broccoli, onions, and carrots
>
> 1½ cups cooked jasmine brown rice
>
> 2 cups baby spinach
>
> 2 teaspoons fat-free vinaigrette dressing
>
> 1 tablespoon nutritional yeast flakes
>
> 1 orange

Dinner:

> 2+ cups mixed red potatoes and sweet potatoes
>
> ½ cup curry vindaloo lentils
>
> 1½ cups stir-fry with green beans, onions, and roasted red bell peppers
>
> 1 cup cherries

 Just because my sample day is listed as three meals doesn't mean you should eat three meals a day. Some days I eat three meals, but on others, I eat seven or eight times. Whether you eat 3 or 12 times a day doesn't matter. When you're a body-managed eater with a whole-food, plant-based, low-fat diet, your hunger and fullness are your trusted guides.

Here's how the servings came out on this particular day:

> **Veggies:** 9 servings (8 to 10+ servings)
>
> **Starchies:** 9 servings (8 to 10+ servings)
>
> **Fruit:** 4 servings (3 or 4 servings)
>
> **Beans and legumes:** 1 serving (2+ servings)
>
> **Nuts and seeds:** 1 serving (1 serving, up to 1 ounce a day)

Above all else, keep it simple. As long as you follow these guidelines, you can liberate yourself from measuring madness and free up more time and energy for living.

Remember, you cannot defeat hunger with willpower. Hunger-intensive diets set you up for disaster with uncontrollable cravings, rebound gain, and all the heartache they bring. I did that for about 30 years before I found my diet ideal that allows—no, encourages, invites, and demands—you to eat according to appetite. That means you eat when you're hungry until you're not. And when you're hungry, you do it again. It's one of the hallmarks and benefits of a whole-food, low-fat, plant-based diet.

Good Fats

But what about "healthy" fats? You need them, right? Absolutely. Fats are an essential nutrient, meaning you need to get them from the food you eat. By now, it should come as no surprise that you can get all the essential fats you need from a whole-food, plant-based diet. You don't need to squeeze the oil out of fiber-rich nuts, seeds, olives, or coconuts. Remember the information on calorie concentration in your food? A prime example of lots of calories that take up a tiny amount of space in your stomach is vegetable oil. At 120 calories per tablespoon and about 4,000 calories per pound, oil occupies very little space and weight in your stomach, at high calorie cost—a *very* high calorie cost.

I know what you're thinking. You're more satisfied after a richer meal that's higher in fat than after a meal that isn't, that having fat in your meals "stabilizes" your appetite for the rest of the day. Sorry, but the research doesn't bear it out. In study after study, comparisons of subjects who ate a high-fat meal compared to those who ate a low-fat, high-carbohydrate meal (given the same number of overall calories in that meal) found that the subjects who ate the higher-fat meal ate more calories at subsequent meals than those who ate a low-fat meal.

You can get ample fat from whole-food sources and, at the same time, reap the fiber, phytonutrient, antioxidant, vitamin, and mineral rewards, too. The best way to obtain essential fats is through legumes, small amounts of nuts, seeds, and even leafy green vegetables. Foods like avocados and olives also provide fat and are superior to oils, which are processed and fiber-free, according to Julieanna Hever, RD, in *The Complete Idiot's Guide to Plant-Based Nutrition*.

For example, in a study reported by J. Cotton and team in the *Journal of Human Nutrition and Diet* in 2007, normal-weight subjects in the Human Appetite Research Unit were served one of three breakfasts. Researchers were interested in tracking hunger intensity and fullness to detect whether the differences in satiety and calories consumed over the course of the rest of the day were any different depending on whether subjects had a high-fat or a low-fat meal. Researchers measured the calories and nutrients the test subjects consumed at lunch and dinner when given the opportunity to eat as much as they wanted, according to their appetite. For the rest of the day until after breakfast the next day, the subjects' food intake was carefully measured.

The test breakfasts consisted of a basic 440-kilocalorie meal for all three groups. One group then was fed an added meal supplement of 362 kilocalories of added fat. Another group was fed an added 362 kilocalories of added carbohydrate. Although no differences were detected between the effects of the basic breakfasts compared with the fat-supplemented breakfast, the carbohydrate-supplement group experienced suppressed hunger for a period of time after consumption.

In a second experiment, the same team directly tested calorie consumption during the postmeal window. Their conclusion? The carbohydrate-supplemented breakfast suppressed subsequent calorie intake, but the fat-supplemented breakfast did not.

Carbohydrates and fats can produce dramatically different effects on satiety. Under these experimental conditions, the fat supplement resulted in no detectable effect on appetite. With these results, it's easy to see how dietary fat can lead to calorie overconsumption.

Some foods can more easily contribute to satiety than others. Calorie charts do not reflect this ultraimportant dimension of the food you eat, which is why studies examining the effects of foods have on "feelings of fullness" can be so helpful. Fruits, vegetables, and starchy vegetables have the highest satiety values, along with beans, lentils, pasta, rice, and whole-grain cereals. Pastries, cakes, and processed sugar-on-fat-on-sugar edibles have the lowest satiety values. That's why that croissant and double-mocha whatever at breakfast, although extremely calorific, doesn't carry you through the day as its calorie count might promise. What a rip.

This means you can just add those fat calories coming along for the ride in that chunk of cheese, slice of meat, or fish filet or whatever fast-food sandwich to all the other calories you've eaten during the day as a bonus energy pack destined for storage. They don't add enough to your satiety to make them worth it, yet they do add easily to your fat stores.

That big bowl of oatmeal for breakfast, on the other hand, is the fast-track to your favorite skinny jeans.

Dealing with Food Cravings

If they're not good for us and just make us fat, why do these high-fat, high-sugar foods appeal to us so much? It doesn't seem fair, does it?

I figure our bodies do everything for a reason. Biologically speaking, we are programmed to survive. High-fat, high-sugar foods are the best thing you can eat to add new fat stores and protect the ones you already have, thus ensuring your survival.

 According to Neal Barnard, MD, in *Breaking the Food Seduction,* when high-fat, high-sugar, processed, and flavor-enhanced foods are in the vicinity—even just in the mind's eye or your memory—a whole cascade of biochemicals is activated, driving you to indulge.

Add to this the incredibly complex flavor traps food manufacturers add to such foods, and it's no wonder we're playing with a handicap. We may have a biological circuitry designed to maintain a balance of energy that keeps us at our ideal healthy weight, but that doesn't often stand up in the face of easy access to foods high in additives that give us an overpowering push to eat. Food manufacturers know this. They add sugar, fat, and salt that make you want to eat more, in spite of your better judgment. This hijacks your pleasure hormones, even in anticipation of the stimulation, rendering you helpless. It's not a character flaw; it's your survival biology kicking in. It's not your fault.

Plus—and this is huge—if you chronically undereat, hunger will build so you're unable to resist the pull of these foods. You end up giving in to the cookies and the pint (or more) of premium. And according to Jean Antonello in *How to Become Naturally Thin by Eating More,* considering hunger is a primary stress, is it any wonder you cave and pig out on all the foods least compatible with your weight-loss goals? You're not an emotional overeater; you're just hungry.

Secrets for Success

With the freedom of being a plant-based eater at your own healthy and trim weight—which you will become when you implement the instructions of my simple food plan—comes responsibility. You knew there was a catch! Settle down. We're just talking about a little plan-ahead smarts. It multiplies your currency in a job easily done.

Always Be Prepared

If your plan is to eat a healthy lunch of soup, a big salad, and a veggie sandwich, it doesn't help if all that's within reach is the double-cheese pizza your coworkers ordered for lunch. When you aren't prepared with the food you need to support your health, you're faced with options that are likely not in your plan, which you'll have little willpower to resist when you're so hungry that your biological urge to overcome the stress of your grumbling stomach overrides your better judgment. Before you know it, you're off with the rest of them on a high-fat, high-calorie, low-fiber ride.

It's essential that you always be prepared. After all, you can't eat what you don't have.

And if you think getting to the market, stocking your fridge, and packing and preparing your lunches is inconvenient, remember this: it's far less inconvenient than being hungry and fat at the same time.

Leveling the Playing Field

Being an eat-according-to-your-appetite eater demands that you level the playing field of what's on your plate. That's why you need an understanding of satiation, satiety, and how concentrated the calories are in the foods you eat. And that's why eating within the five food groups is the answer to your health and weight dilemma.

 If you don't understand why processed, fiber-free, and high-fat foods are the problem, you'll be stuck continuously fighting a war with hunger you'll never win.

With a whole-food, plant-based, low-fat diet, you can trust your hunger and fullness signals to keep you at your trimmest. The reason we've become fat in the first place is because we count on our food to keep our appetite satisfied. But now we know that unless the foods you choose are bringing hunger satisfaction without excess calories, you're going to continue to play hide-and-seek with hunger and a leaner body.

This is my number-one objection to the "intuitive eating" movement, in which you eat what sounds good or what your body craves because your body must be telling you you're lacking in some essential nutrient that food contains.

Here's my counter rule to "intuitive eating": true nutritional need comes in the form of hunger for real food, not cravings. If you're craving chocolate or doughnuts or a pint of double-chunk whatever, you need to find out whether you're hungry or really just interested in a taste pleasure cycle or stress break. Does an apple or a sandwich appeal? If not, you can be sure of one of two things: either you are so overly hungry that your body is looking for the most energy-dense food available to boost your survival quotient, or you're not feeling hunger and the craving is for the stress-relieving chemical cascade that's released when you eat that triple-mocha whatever. Or both.

Potatoes Are Plants, Too

Remember the role starchies play in hunger satisfaction and the long-term satiety that your goal of being well fed without being fat demands. If, in your mind's eye, "plant-based" conjures up pictures of only leafy green veggies and carrot sticks, you need to change that image right now. Include a robust starch section in your diet. Don't make the mistake I did of hedging on the role these comfort foods play in keeping you slim, healthy, and happy. You were meant for each other.

Case in point, if you need a little push: in a 1979 study reported by O. Mickelson and team in the *American Journal of Clinical Nutrition*, a group of overweight men was given the dietary directive to make only one change to their diet: adding 12 slices of bread a day. That's right, 12 pieces of bread each day. No additional exercise was added, and no foods were purposely eliminated. Over the course of 8 weeks, these men lost an average of $7\frac{1}{2}$ pounds. That's about 1 pound a week—just by eating more bread (not, however, bread dipped in olive oil or slathered with butter). Evidently, when eaten with meals, the bread provided increased gastric stretch and weight, naturally and painlessly replacing some of the calories the subjects usually ate.

Crowding Out the Compromises

It's time to incorporate more foods that are compatible with your health and weight-loss goals. When you eat oats for breakfast, for example, you crowd out fiber-free pastries, cottage cheese, eggs, and high-fat bacon. When you mound hummus on your whole-grain bread for lunch, you nudge out the high-fat, highly concentrated calories from the highly energy-dense mayonnaise. When you make a simple bean burger and baked potato fries for dinner, you replace the beef and french fries. Think of the foods you love that might take just a few tweaks to fit them in your new way of eating.

Remember, when your diet is full of high-fat, high-sugar food or processed products, you are at a weight-management handicap. Your stomach doesn't register "full"—that is, satiation—until quite possibly long after your calorie needs have been met. This makes it difficult to reduce your body's current fat stores and easily invites even more fat storage.

 Refined, processed, and fiber-free foods present tremendous challenges to your weight as a direct result of the calorie shift real food undergoes when it's folded, bend, spindled, or otherwise altered in processing and refining. Remember, just because it's edible doesn't mean you should eat it.

Eating Enough Calories

Being low in calories doesn't make a food automatically "good," any more than being high calories makes a food "bad." If you get carried away with eating too many low-calorie foods, chances are, you'll hit the hunger wall. That's what's happened to me.

You won't be completely satisfied with a stomach full of "rabbit food" without some of the more calorific starchy vegetables and whole grains. It's the combination of these foods that provides satiety and gives you a better chance of getting and staying healthy and trim. Following the guidelines of hunger satisfaction means you must respect all of them, just like the three pillars of fitness success. If you don't, your hunger drive will kick in as cravings and blindside you. Every time.

Opting for Complex Carbs

A refresher course on carbs is in order. When we eat them as whole foods, carbohydrates come right along with their nutrient buddies such as fiber, fats, and protein and are presented in a way our bodies were designed to eat. Remember, we eat food, not isolated macronutrients. So for conversation's sake, let's focus on foods that get the highest percentage of their calories from carbohydrates: grains and starchy vegetables.

The more complex and therefore less processed carbohydrates are, the lower they are in energy density and the higher their satiation and satiety value for you. This makes complex carbohydrates your new best friend. Whole grains (such as brown rice, oats, wheat, and quinoa), as well as starchy vegetables (like yams, winter squash, sweet potatoes, corn and peas, and beans and legumes) should form the calorie base of your healthy, plant-based diet.

 Not all carbs are created equal. When considering the most highly refined carbohydrates made from low-fiber grains that have been finely ground into flour and baked into crackers and pastries, remember that the calorie concentration of carbohydrate foods climbs, bowl for bowl, the more a whole food is processed and distanced from its original state. This processing increases the surface area of these foods, resulting in absorption of a higher number of calories, as reported by G. Haber and team in *Lancet,* 1977, and K. Heaton in *The American Journal of Clinical Nutrition,* 1988. It's easy to overeat these foods because their taste can be so tempting. If your goal is weight loss, stick to whole grains and save these processed foods for rare occasions.

That said, there's no need to obsess about each bite you take. I've had occasion to travel to far-flung corners of the planet where I could find not a single grain of brown rice, and the only options I could eat with my veggies for a week or two were white rice and noodles. But because I was vigilant about not letting those calorie-concentrated fats find their way onto my plate, and because fiber-free animal products are always off my menu, I've done just fine—and sometimes I've even come back trimmer. That's eating freedom.

Every day, I'm thrilled to walk into my kitchen, happily armed with the knowledge that I have shelves of beautiful, delicious foods to choose from, foods I can eat to my heart's—and my stomach's—content. I know now from years of experience that this way of eating not only keeps me healthy and well fed, but also keeps me trim. I never tire of being able to buy cartfuls of whole foods wherever in the world I happen to be, cook and eat the way I do at home, and easily keep my shape with the simple activities I enjoy, be it hiking, walking, doing a few Fit Quickies, or engaging in other elements of play. When you get the food right, the fitness is so much easier. It's a wonderful way to live.

Getting Started with Plant-Based Eating

Whether you've been enjoying a plant-based diet for some time and want to make it healthier or tweak it for weight loss, or you're just beginning to wrap your head around the idea of plant-based eating and are excited to get going, the answer to the question "How do I get started?" is the same. Start where you are. Take an honest look at where you are now, compared to where you want to be.

If you've been stuck but now can see that you may be a few adjustments away from your ideal, healthy weight, you probably already see where you can make some simple yet beneficial shifts. On the other hand, if it seems like you have so far to go to get where want to be, relax, take a breath, and remember that every journey is completed by placing one foot in front of the other—or, in this case, eating one meal at a time.

Keep it simple, and try to focus on what you want to eat. It's less important to get in X number of servings of beans a day, for example, than to find a diet full of foods you can actually see yourself eating for the rest of your life. Opt for food that leaves you feeling full, satisfied, and energized.

 Remember, don't eat only vegetables in an attempt to lose weight fast. That can create more problems than it solves. It's very, very important not to go hungry. Be free with starches. I'd rather you err on the side of too much when getting started, to offset carbophobia, which tends to linger and threatens your success. I encourage you to reread my story to boost your confidence. In the words of John McDougall, MD, in *The Starch Solution,* "Enjoyment and satisfaction are the keys to successful diet change and weight loss."

What's Already Working?

Pastas, grain and vegetable dishes, chili and cornbread, potatoes and salad, and oatmeal with fruit are all familiar favorites, as are sandwiches, soups, burritos, and wraps. These foods are all easy to prepare and include in a whole-food, plant-based diet. Swap in beans for beef, balsamic for oil-based dressing, and vegetable stock–braised vegetables for fried. Sit down and make a list of all your favorite dishes, and then get creative coming up with alternatives to any calorie-concentrated, fiber-deficient animal product ingredients.

Here are a few ideas to get you started:

- Pasta with meat sauce is now pasta with marinara sauce.

- Chili is now *bean* chili, without the meat.

- Taco night is now … taco night, with veggie refried beans (no need for oil—just mash them up), tomatoes, lettuce, onions, salsa, and corn.

- Sandwiches are now … sandwiches, with whole-grain bread and hummus or other mashed bean spread, grated carrots, sliced tomatoes and onions, and even potatoes or sweet potatoes mixed in with the other veggies and mustard for spice. The sandwich story really takes on new dimensions when you think outside the baloney box. And no need to sigh your way through a meager open-faced sandwich on "diet" bread. Go for the gusto with a full-on sammy.

- Burger night is now … veggie burger night! These are easy to make at home with beans, whole grains, and chopped onions, garlic, and other spicy veggies. Or simply grill a portobello mushroom for an easy, savory, and delicious solution.

The ease and simplicity of preparation are found in repeated patterns. Notice that my meals are built around a basic structure within which ingredients rotate and change. Whether I'm eating grains and veggies, potatoes and salad, or soup, I vary the kinds of beans or lentils I use, the variety of potatoes I bake, the color of the chopped vegetables in the salad, and the kind and color of the grains I cook. You don't have to get fancy with a long list of recipes—unless, of course, you want to!

Strategizing with Small Steps or Big Leaps

Next, consider a strategy to help you move forward. Some people do well with a "boot camp" approach—immersion in a set of principles for a certain period of time. This strategy has proven to be successful over and over again in my programs. It can bring rapid results, build confidence, and give you a good shot at resetting your tastes for new fare. However, it is not without its risks, especially if you're going it alone and living in a sea of standard American diet eaters. It can be done, but don't leave it to chance and assume that you'll be "in the mood" to make good choices. Preparation is a prerequisite. You need to anticipate and be ready, consider all the variables and possibilities for derailment, and find as many avenues of support as you can.

Others build long-term success by using the immersion method while being selective and single-minded about exactly what they're immersing themselves in. This one-step-at-a-time method is a practical and prudent approach, and it's a strategy suggested by Doug Lisle, PhD, an expert of habit change. You select one thing to add, do differently, or change for a certain period of time. You select something that's moving you in the direction you want to go, something that's a bit of a stretch, yet in your heart and head you affirm, "Yeah, I could do that!" Raise the bar, but don't set it so high that it's out of reach.

For example, pick something to add to your diet every day for a week, such as a big bowl of oatmeal or other whole-grain cereal at breakfast, or a serving of beans at lunch. Every day. By week's end, if 5 out of 7 days you have a star on the chart next to your chosen objective, you've got a win, a mission accomplished, a new sense of confidence, and an improvement in your health. And then add something else.

If you didn't accomplish your objective for most of the week, it's time to reassess. Were you prepared with what you needed every day? How can you support yourself for greater success next week? If your mission to have oatmeal every day faltered, would preparing your oats to soak overnight in a pot on the stove help you be more ready in the morning? You bet it would.

 In addition to what you put on your plate, take time to reflect on your eating behaviors. If you're caught in cycles of under- and overeating, you need to take a look at something besides *what* you're eating. Addressing eating *behaviors* along with the food has been essential to my success, and it may well be for you, too. Undereating leads to overeating.

Keep building on your success. Be a compassionate taskmaster, but expect to fall short on occasion. That's okay. As time progresses, you'll have made substantial gains in crowding out less desirable foods. Imagine what you can accomplish in 6 months or a year! Take the long view, and picture your future success.

As another example, you may decide to eat a hearty bowl of soup full of vegetables and beans every day. Here's the perfect opportunity to cook once for several days' worth of meals. This is one of my healthy habits. I cut up onions, carrots, celery, sweet potato or potato, a head of kale, and any other vegetables I'm in the mood for, and cook it all in the pressure cooker for 2 minutes. Then I add some big scoops of beans or lentils and season with vegetable broth. Sometimes I add barley, rice, or other whole grains, too. Talk about hearty! A bowl of this at lunch satisfies like you wouldn't believe. Even when you're ready and hungry for the next meal, your appetite will be still be satisfied. Soup loaded with veggies and chock full of starches and beans is a weight-loss winner.

If you're a veteran vegan looking for an answer to why your weight and health might be stuck, I'm betting you now know why. Just because it's vegetarian or vegan doesn't mean it's healthy. And no matter where you are on the food and eating continuum, to advance, you need the advantage of motivation. Perfect timing for mastery of mind-set.

MOTIVATION AND MIND-SET FOR SUCCESS

"I just can't seem to get up and do *anything*. I know I need to—and I want to—but just can't get the mind-set."

"I have good intentions but don't follow through, either with eating or with exercise."

"I need help getting into a routine and sticking with it. I have times, even during one day, when I fall off the wagon. There's always an excuse."

"Exercise motivation is my big problem, and I have trouble sticking to a fitness plan."

"Tackling the last 10 pounds and sticking to an eating plan for more than a few days is challenging as frustrations set in. Impatience is my middle name, and I give in quickly when I don't see immediate results. I need help with a better positive mental outlook."

"I'm good at eating healthy. But I have a hard time fitting exercise into my schedule. I know I need to make it a priority, but somehow I don't."

Do any of these sound like you? If so, you're not alone. While preparing this book, I conducted several surveys asking people about their biggest health, fitness, and weight-loss challenges. Responses about staying motivated to exercise or eat right were at the top of the list.

Maybe all you need to achieve your healthy fitness goals is a good food plan. Perhaps getting some solid answers about exercise and a workout system is all that's necessary to tip you into the success circle. But what if you find you still can't seem to get it together consistently enough to realize your fitness dreams?

After years of disheartening stop-and-start weight-loss attempts and lasting success always just out of my reach, you might wonder what made the difference for me. What changed so I could finally not only lose the weight, but easily keep it off while enjoying a healthy, happy relationship with food, eating, and my body? If that extra step—the third pillar of the three foundations of sound exercise, healthy diet, and a winning mind-set about it all—eludes you, keeps you running in circles, and seems to sabotage your success, this chapter is for you.

You can have the best exercise and diet plans in the world, but if you don't use them to your benefit, they're worthless. The way I see it, there are two main problems here: staying motivated and getting out of your own way. The allure of a better body gets you ramped up for change, only to fizzle with the early obstacles that kick you out of a new, healthy groove. Or you start to have some measure of success, only to find old, familiar habits hijacking your progress. Or maybe you're doing fine on the new plan and you just get bored. Where's that part of you that knows how to follow through?

Change Your Mind, Change Your Body, Change Your Life

Is it possible that what makes the difference is a simple yet pivotal shift in your thinking? I think so, especially when you have the tools of exercise and eating on your side for leverage. The question, then, is how do you progress from the patterns of thinking that keep you locked in a spiral of limited progress—or what can seem like desperately painful lack of progress.

I'm going to share some powerful tools for constructing your mind-set for change. With these insights and instructions into small shifts of thinking, you can achieve astonishing results.

I want you to see that these shifts, rather than being one big breakthrough that delivers the answer, instead are each doable actions that, together with your exercise and eating plan, will transform your life. When an airplane shifts off course by a fraction of a degree, it can land in an entirely different location than if it had stayed on its flight plan. Think of the results you're getting right now as your flight plan. All it takes is a few nudges of what you eat, how you move, and how you think—onto a new course—and you open the opportunity to landing in an entirely different place. Small shifts can result in big change.

Each time you make a choice, you are one step closer to solidifying a habit. Habits in themselves aren't a bad thing. They can lead to a lifetime of radiant success … or one of frustration and bad health. Quite quickly, your habits become your lifestyle, day after day, year after year. Your challenge for change is as simple as changing your choices.

So how do you do it? How do you navigate the roller coaster of commitment and the stress that takes you off track and end up with more wins than setbacks? Can you really change course? How do you find your voice of focus, your compelling commitment, the "Just do it!" in you? How do you reach the part of you connected with your better judgment and inspired to realize your greater potential and higher ideals?

If you're like many people, you'll do just about anything to stay in your comfort zone. After all, you're *comfortable* there. Yet if you want change, if you want to accomplish anything, you have to move *out* of that zone and onto a new flight path. And that starts with what's going on in your head.

Choices, Habits, Lifestyle, Destiny

Just like physical habits, you have mental habits —good and bad. When you address your thought habits, you open the door to thinking differently.

It's absolutely possible to revolutionize your responses and especially the actions you take. When you face the obstacles to your success—those obvious obstacles and those that lie hidden just under the surface, blindsiding you— you move more confidently toward your goals.

If you feel uncomfortable when in transition to healthier diet and exercise, take it as a good sign. It shows you're nudging yourself out of your comfort zone and onto a new course. If you want something different from what you've been getting, you need to *do* something different.

Expect a learning curve. Expect the shoe to pinch a little while you break it in. Expect and allow for the need to plan and organize in support of your new direction. Expect some setbacks mixed in with the wins. Change for healthy fitness and weight loss doesn't happen in a straight line. Expect that you'll need to adjust your tools of navigation from time to time. Remember, journeys to improvement, especially when we have to shift our way of doing something, often have rises and dips in the road. It's going to take focus, imagination, commitment, compassion, heart, and learning to ride the wave.

It's about intention and taking action by making different choices, one choice at a time. You already know the basics of what to do each week for healthy fitness. You already know the ideal diet for health and weight loss. Puttering around and pretending you don't keeps you cemented in your current behaviors—and the same results—whether those behaviors are habits of thinking, exercise, diet, or thought.

 Your choices become your habits. Your habits become your lifestyle. And what does your lifestyle become? Your destiny.

"Choices, habits, lifestyle, destiny"—this was a big breakthrough phrase for me. Make it your new mantra. There's no time like now. Your health, weight, and fitness are fundamental to leading a vibrant, energetic, and productive life—a life filled with confidence in your body that brings you more fully into expression, living your potential, pursuing your passions, and realizing your dreams.

Even if you know what you need to change, if you don't have the drive of purpose behind it, it can too easily get lost in the din of daily life. It's just part of the human predicament. It takes a plan for smart eating and exercise, of course, but it also takes attention to mind-set mastery, of learning how to focus.

Finding Your *What* and Your *Why*

If you don't have a vision of what you want to be, what you want to create with your health, fitness, and body ideal, this is a big part of your problem. You need a *what* and a *why*. How can you expect to stay motivated when you're unclear about what you want in the first place? When you take an honest look and clean up some of the chaos surrounding the indecision of where you want to go, your ability to focus becomes easier. If you already have an idea of what you want, you're ahead of the game.

The Importance of Imagination

They say the real secret to change—the solid kind of change you might be seeking with losing weight, changing your diet, or improving your shape—starts with the belief that you'll succeed. You've got to think it's possible and imagine yourself successful, or you won't get more than one foot out the door, let alone down any of the steps that get you where you want to go.

But you have to take it a step further. *Belief is not enough.* For me, one of the most important agents of change was allowing myself to imagine how it would feel to be healthy, fit, and slender—*now*. Try it for yourself. Imagine what it would be like if you didn't have a "weight problem" or "body problem." Imagine it, and step right into that thought as a reality. Now imagine what your consciousness would be like without the layer of self-limitation and burden because you're "too fat," "too out of shape," or "too *whatever*."

Playing with these concepts can be exhilarating and frightening at the same time. But don't back away! When you allow in the insights that come from imagination, they are, ultimately, unbelievably transforming. Persist in trying this new attitude. It will reveal valuable pieces of information. This exercise led me to three enlightening breakthroughs; maybe you'll recognize yourself here, too:

- It made me realize how much tension I had built up around food and eating.

- It drove home the futility—and absurdity—of continuing to see myself as someone fat and with a weight problem while expecting any real change in my weight.

- It showed me how much of my identity was wrapped up in this ongoing struggle.

These breakthroughs still didn't make me thin—not right then, anyway. But realizing them was a big step.

And here's something you must really believe. Highlight, circle, underline, or write 100 times the following:

> You must change your mind before you can change your body. *You* control your flight plan.

If your head and heart are stuck in a rut of past failures and frustrations, that's where you'll stay, as much as you might think you want to get out. If your focus is on the difficulties and impossibilities of change, how can you expect to achieve it? To really experience change, you need to address these points:

- You must give up identification with past failure.

- You must embrace the ability to see yourself succeeding.

This might sound challenging, but believe me, it's not impossible. *You* are the agent of change. *You* are the magic bullet.

Commitment: Key Strategies to Change

Three key strategies are instrumental in starting the process of change. You must seriously address them, or you needn't bother wasting your time trying to lose weight, change your health, or improve your shape. They're *that* important.

Here they are:

Abstain from worrying about your present shape. Worrying about your current condition and anxiety about the distance you have to travel to your health, weight-loss, or body-shaping goal only magnifies your doubt and clouds your vision. You end up feeling uncertain, negative, and filled with self-doubt. You second-guess your goals and your ability to realize them. Yet certainty, clarity, and confidence, even if you aren't feeling them every moment, are reachable through the power of your imagination.

Look where you're going instead of where you've been. Wasting time and energy worrying about your present shape is just that—wasting time and energy. Instead, focus on your devotion to your daily objectives, the specific actions you take every day, that will bring you, one step at a time, to what you're creating for your future. Cultivate the vision of you at your personal best.

Identify with accomplishment and success. Think back to a time when you were successful in something in your life. Any accomplishment that comes to mind works. Step fully into that feeling of success, of winning, no matter what the realm. Own it. Bask in it. *This is the winner you can be—and are.* This is a very, very important part of the cultivation of your vision.

Now take it a step further. Ask yourself the following questions:

- What did you do to achieve that important accomplishment?

- What steps did you take to make it happen?

- What qualities did you demonstrate that resulted in your success? Tenacity? Courage? Organization?

Did you make a plan, work toward it, create an attitude of devotion toward your cause, and keep the vision of accomplishing your goal in front of you, even when it got challenging or you experienced setbacks? The very same things you did then are what you're going to draw upon now to move toward your new success with your health, fitness, and weight.

Winning Qualities

Winners have three key qualities:

Winners— in any venue—don't wallow in their past failures. They don't ignore or suppress them; they just acknowledge them and redirect their energy to the effort and preparation that keep moving them forward.

Winners don't focus on how many times they've fallen; they just get up again. Your keywords are *practice* and *redirect*. When you notice yourself focusing on your falls, make a note of it, and look for steps to make a different choice. Remember the flight path analogy.

Winners don't say things like, "I can't do this." This language reinforces failure. Where did we get these ideas about ourselves? (More about that in a minute.) It's time you found a new way to frame your objectives.

Practice the qualities of a winner. Think of them as three big engines powering your success.

Accomplishment and Success Activity

Take time this week to sit down with pen and paper to answer the questions raised in the "Commitment: Key Strategies to Change" section. Think back to a success from your past. Again, it needn't be huge, but it needs to be something you achieved after challenging yourself *by reaching beyond who you were before*.

In your notes, write detailed answers to these questions:

- What did you do to achieve this important accomplishment, and what steps did you take to make it happen?

- Did you make a plan, work toward it, create an attitude of devotion toward that cause, and keep a vivid mental picture of accomplishing that goal in front of you?

- What qualities did you demonstrate that resulted in your success? Tenacity? Courage? Organization?

Then each day this week, make a conscious effort to practice the three key strategies to change.

> Remember the key strategies to change: abstain from worrying about your present shape, look where you're going instead of where you've been, and identify with and feel the emotions of accomplishment and success.

The Problem: Self-Sabotage

You don't know what you don't know about your fears, thoughts, feelings, and self-sabotaging beliefs. These are the hidden obstacles to your success. Yet how you think about yourself and your abilities is simply that—how you *think* about yourself. Your thoughts—or more precisely, your responses to them—are largely habits.

Think about it. On any given day, you can have the same experience someone with a different life background and history has, but you could have an entirely different thought and emotional response. It's just your habit to respond as you do. And you can change your habits.

Negative Self-Talk

Negative self-talk is a bad habit. Do you frequently hear yourself saying any of the following?

> "I'll never lose weight because …."

> "It's impossible to resist eating …."

> "I won't be able to deal with …."

> "I'll never be able to …."

> "I'll never be able to give up …."

> "I can't work out late in the day."

This type of negative self-talk diminishes your self-confidence. It creates a spiral of feeling and action that hold you hostage.

Self-Fulfilling Thought Patterns

Your thoughts (which, remember, are just that … thoughts), create feelings that move you to action (remember, inaction is an action, too), and from that you get results. Repeated practice of the sequence cements the pattern, and it becomes a self-fulfilling process. Until you decide you're going to go through the discomfort of dislodging that pattern from its well-worn groove, you're doomed. (Or *liberated*, depending on what kind of patterns you build going forward.)

If for years, maybe even decades, you've had repeated failures to reach your health and weight-loss goals, these hidden obstacles are probably creating sticking points. Intellectually, this makes sense. Yet when you really experience and face these blocks, an awakening happens after which you'll never be quite the same.

Examine this list of ways you might be sabotaging your behaviors with habituated thought patterns (adapted from Fabienne Frederickson's *Mindset Retreat*, 2011):

- Do you often make excuses for not taking consistent action to raise your level of health and fitness?

- Do you have a habit of focusing on what's lacking instead of on what you want?

- Do you hang on to a very limited idea of how much control you can really have on your health and fitness, making it a convenient crutch?

- Do you allow fear of rejection and failure to get in the way of taking action? Why take a risk by going for what you want or wearing what you want? What will they think?

- Do you resent attractive, slim people?

- Are you putting too much focus on the negative influence in your surroundings, especially when you don't feel family or friends are supportive?

- Are you honestly willing to do what it takes to change your health, weight, shape, or *whatever?*

- Are you compelled to compare your progress to others'?

- Are you clear on why you want to improve your body and how having health and vitality will make you even more fully expressive? Or is it too scary?

- Are you reluctant—afraid, even—to invest in yourself? Do you have a nagging sense that you shouldn't spend time or money on *you?*

- Are you indecisive? Perhaps you don't always trust yourself to make the right decision, so no decision often feels like the better option. Or you make a decision on where you want to go with your diet or exercise, only to jump ship in a few days when the next bright, shiny object catches your eye.

- Do you procrastinate, often using perfectionism as your excuse?

- Secretly, do you wonder whether you can truly handle success? Are you afraid of what people will think of you if you do begin to succeed?

When challenging yourself to change, you'll discover these fears, thoughts, and beliefs aren't necessarily valid. That doesn't mean you don't experience them as real and deal with all the fallout from engaging with them. But they're not permanent. They can change—*you* can change them.

The longer you continue to reinforce belief in these erroneous ideas, even on a subconscious level, the longer it will take to achieve the health and fitness freedom you really want. Every thought you have creates a feeling within you that dictates your actions. Each action then creates a particular result in your life. A limiting thought—even just one—creates a negative feeling that prevents you from taking action that then impacts your results.

Where did this all come from, anyway? Where did these thoughts first get seeded, only to grow into huge, unmanageable weeds? The beliefs and fears that sabotage you from reaching success come from a variety of different places:

- Hand-me-down beliefs from parents, other relatives, and friends

- Cultural or social expectations

- Childhood experiences, real and imagined

- Beliefs friends and acquaintances hold as "truths" that, in your heart of hearts, are not yours

- The media

These influences are all around you, and it can seem impossible to claim your independence from them. But changing your habituated cycles of thoughts and their results is crucial if you want to realize your healthy weight goal, have a fit body, and have a healthy and *happy* relationship with both.

The "What the Hell" Effect

There's a phenomenon psychologists call the "what the hell" effect. You can probably guess what this hidden (or not-so-hidden) obstacle is without my even having to explain it—we all recognize it instantly.

The "what the hell" effect is the most common reason people give up on goals. As explained by McGonigal in *The Willpower Instinct*, when you set huge goals for yourself, expecting 24-hour turnaround to a new you, you set yourself up to fail. You can't become a completely transformed person overnight. When you trip up or fall short, even in a small way, you figure "Oh, what the hell. I'm never going to change. I broke my diet. It's all over so I might as well go back to the way things were."

Setting smaller, more realistic goals—goals that incrementally yet powerfully rechart your course—builds success, one win at a time. And believe it or not, expecting some trip-ups along the way helps. People who accept that being less than perfect is part of the process are far more likely to succeed in the long term. Setting smaller, specific goals and steps to inch you forward, as well as having compassion for yourself when you do slip up, pacifies those occasions you don't quite reach your goal—those times when your actions come up against the voice that has your better interests at heart. Respecting both of these drives with compassion for yourself disarms the agents of self-destruction.

The Antidote to Negative Thought Patterns

The antidote to negative thought pattern spirals is to interrupt the thought pattern and set yourself on a new trajectory. You can't control thoughts and feelings as they arise. But you can learn new strategies to change your response to those thoughts and feelings, derailing previous patterns so you can get out of a rut and into a new groove.

Actions bring the powerful sense of accomplishment into play and boost your self-confidence.

Learning to Ride the Wave

It may sound obvious, but for me, understanding this was one of the biggest breakthroughs to my success: just because thoughts and feelings surface doesn't mean you have to react with the same, often inappropriate responses you've always had. You can change your actions to a direction that builds your success instead of tearing it down.

Research tells us the best way to deal with thoughts we don't want to think or feelings we don't want to feel is to just accept that they happen. Acknowledge that you don't have control over whether a thought or emotion comes up, and realize that the harder you try to push away a thought or feeling, the stronger its influence becomes.

Here's where the shift happens, though: even if you can't control what comes into your mind, you don't need to focus and ruminate on it. Start to see these thoughts, memories, and emotions that come up like a wave that rises, crests, and then subsides on its own. You don't suppress it, push it away, dive into it, or otherwise interact with it. You just watch the wave and wait it out. S. Bowen and A. Martlett also call it "surfing the urge" in their 2009 report in the *Psychology of Addictive Behavior*. You don't suppress it, push it away, dive into it, or otherwise get enmeshed. You "watch the wave" and you just wait it out. Brilliant!

Instead of fantasizing that you're going to completely change who you are, what you think, or what emotions you're going to eliminate, or magically morph into something different, simply accept that you can't control some obstacles. The less you try to control them, the more they lose their power and influence.

 A technique that taught me how to "watch the wave" is insight meditation, a very direct and simple process of just being present in your body. It defuses stress and brings calm, explores the mind-body relationship, expands your sense of who you are beyond your fears and self-judgment, and awakens your capacity for insight and wisdom. Practice the meditation or centering technique of your choice; I can't recommend this highly enough.

Practicing New Thoughts

When you become more aware of that space between a thought arising and your habit of response to that thought, you can create a different comeback. It's a moment of intervention, a door to an alternate route.

Take time this week to sit and quickly list at least five beliefs you've inherited from your parents, teachers, friends, or social circle. Next to each of these beliefs, write an "alternate route" describing another possible way of thinking about that same thing.

For example:

> **Belief:** I'm afraid to speak in front of a group because I might be embarrassed.
>
> **Alternate route:** Many people learn to overcome their shyness to speak to groups and enjoy it. So could I.
>
> **Belief:** Thin, fit people are vain.
>
> **Alternate route:** Slim, fit people often are people who care about their health and energy and who make healthy eating and sufficient activity a priority.

Viewing "thinking" as a choice—just a way of thinking we have learned and practiced over and over again—can be quite liberating. You learn you literally can change your mind—and change your body, and change your life.

Finding the Big in the Small

Along the way to your long-term goals, acknowledge your benchmarks. For example, if you have a long-term goal of losing 40 pounds, you know it's not going to come all at once. It'll come in chunks of 1, and 2, and 10 pounds. Each of these increments is a benchmark, an opportunity to celebrate and reinforce your progress. This celebrating and reinforcing creates momentum. They might seem like small steps, but they're the brickwork of your big win. They're the big in the small.

Start with the smallest step, one that's a very specific intention, like eating a big bowl of oatmeal and fruit for breakfast. Research suggests that when you set a *specific* intention, you're much more likely to follow through with it. And the smaller the intention, the more likely you are to have a successful experience, which makes it more likely that you'll continue setting goals.

You can build many positive points into your day to provide increased momentum and help you stay focused. Accomplishing your daily objectives, no matter how small they are, is an important incentive. Objectives are the actions you take and choices you make that move you forward toward your long-term goals. For example, here are three examples of daily health and weight-loss objectives you could set:

- Eat a big bowl of whole grains and fruit for breakfast.

- Eat a large salad.

- Move your body.

Never underestimate the importance of each of these seemingly small steps. Completing the necessary little things every day carries you forward to your long-term goals. They're part of your flight plan. Pursue every opportunity you have to let the incentive of checking a key element off your list pull you ahead with momentum. Imagine the possibilities!

The Mysteries of Managing Success

Maybe this has happened to you: you're moving ahead with your health and fitness plan, you've lost a little weight or your clothing fits a little better, and you can tell you're succeeding! Yet somehow you find yourself "celebrating" with all the wrong foods. What's going on here? Why are you doing the opposite of what's giving you the good results you're celebrating?

"Celebrating" with the "wrong" foods is a stress-response habit. What's stressful about losing some weight? Remember, any shakeup of your emotions presents a form of stress. And it doesn't have to be a negative emotion; it can be anything that rattles your equilibrium.

If you find that the shift into success drives you to rich, high-fat, high-sugar foods, potentially three things are going on here:

- You're hungry because you didn't eat enough early in the day, and your body is trying to get your attention so you'll feed it.

- You have the habit of responding to emotional equilibrium disruption by grounding yourself with eating. (Usually preventable by paying attention to the first bullet.)

- Your success is running up against one or more of your limiting beliefs, creating a cognitive dissonance that demands relief. Watch the wave.

That's all the more reason to be sure you eat well, avoid the pitfalls of growing hunger, and protect yourself from stress with stress-management practices such as meditation and exercise. Remember, physical exercise relieves stress and strengthens your brain's executive command center (see the "Winding Up Your Willpower" chapter), enhancing your ability to make choices that are in your best long-term interests.

Focus: Set Priorities and Make Plans

Focus is the most powerful tool you have for maintaining your motivation. If you lose focus—the big *why* of your health and fitness goals—you can be pretty sure your dreams aren't going to come to fruition. It takes a while to establish the new habits of eating, exercise, and thinking necessary for change.

Setting priorities about your health and making plans to follow through with your goals is how you show respect and honor for your higher aspirations.

If you repeatedly let other things get in the way of working out, you're sending yourself the message that your health isn't important. You're saying the daily checklist you need to keep in place to achieve your goals isn't a priority after all.

Being prepared with the healthy food you need to eat to meet your fuel requirements each day is one example of the importance of setting priorities and making plans. Is it inconvenient to pack and prepare a healthy assortment of delicious and filling foods before you leave the house for the day? Is it inconvenient to set out what you need for breakfast the night before what you know will be a rushed morning? Is it inconvenient to take the time to stop at the market at the end of a busy day when you know there's nothing to eat at home? Remember this: *it's not nearly as inconvenient as being fat and hungry at the same time.*

If you keep doing things the way you're doing them, you're going to keep getting what you've been getting. Set your goals, build in the flexibility you know you'll probably need, and get in the habit of keeping promises with yourself.

And keep your goals in front of you. If you find yourself not thinking of your specific goal more than once every few days or every couple weeks, your priorities have definitely slipped—and so will your success. Once you've established an optimal dietary, exercise, rest, and mind-set structure, you also have to plan how you're going to follow through on each part so you create a successful whole.

Life will continue to interrupt and create diversions—and opportunities. Your success depends on being able to manage setbacks and stick to your plan.

Compassion: A Critical Component

Setbacks happen. Most of us believe guilt and remorse is what's going to get us back on track. According to Kelly McGonigal in *The Willpower Instinct*, this is one of the biggest myths about change and willpower. This is probably a carryover from when, as children, we needed to be admonished for something we did so we'd change our behavior. But as adults, apparently guilt and shame motivates us to get back on track far less than we suspect. Research tells us that the harder we are on ourselves after a setback, the more we turn that setback into evidence against ourselves. It goes against all our instincts to say "Everyone makes mistakes."

The evidence says exactly the opposite, however. When you forgive yourself for a setback, remind yourself of what it is you really want, and point yourself back at your goals, you are more successful at getting back on track and reengaging with your goals. When setbacks happen, it's really about forgiving yourself and being that good friend to yourself, reminding yourself what it is you really care about. It's a redirect back onto your flight plan.

Creating new habits of thinking, being, and doing takes ongoing practice. Try thinking of them that way rather than as an endpoint you've achieved; it takes the pressure off. That's why I call motivation and mind-set a practice.

PUTTING IT ALL TOGETHER

In his book, *Mastery: The Keys to Success and Long-Term Fulfillment*, George Leonard brilliantly describes four types of aspirant in any endeavor. The "Dabbler" approaches new pursuits with enormous enthusiasm, often making rapid initial strides. Yet when the inevitable missed mark shows up, the Dabbler figures it's time to dabble in something else. The "Obsessive," also eager for results, thinks it doesn't matter how you get them, as long as you get them fast. Unlike the Dabbler, when brief spurts of progress give way to plateaus, the Obsessive redoubles efforts at the cost of everything else, resulting in burnout. The "Hacker" pursues, skipping initial, critical stages of change, leaving them short on skills for the long haul.

By contrast, door number four, the path of "Mastery," is characterized by practice. It is exemplified by taking simple steps, sometimes steps that might seem quite small. As you hone and polish these steps into skills, they become a scaffold upon which you can build. Mastery respects uneven progress, learning in stages, plateaus, and the need for diligence.

When it comes to your health, you have to assess the territory, decide what you want, make a plan, prepare, and *practice* for your success. Remember, fulfillment demands focus and support. By the way you prepare yourself, you build the most important success network there is. You support yourself in this endeavor of healthy living; conscious eating; and a slimmer, fitter body.

 Just like a big-league baseball player, you control the two critical elements of success: effort and preparation. You may not always be able to control the results on the diamond, but without the team of effort and preparation for the results you desire, you'll simply keep getting what you're currently getting.

Jump in with Both Feet or Tiptoe In?

In preparation for this book, I surveyed, interviewed, and polled hundreds of readers to find out what you thought about how to go about making changes in your exercise, diet, and otherwise healthy-living lifestyle. I asked, "Which approach do you think delivers the best long-term success: tiptoeing into change or jumping in with both feet?" Perhaps it does depend on the individual or personality type. Think back to your own experiences, and you may just find the best match for you.

The responses to my surveys were "jump in with both feet" over the "tiptoe in" approach, at a ratio of about 6:1. Maybe that's just because the "jumpers" are more likely to speak out? We'll never know. A small number of responders said they did "a little of both." For example, if they had jumped into an exercise or dietary change for health at one point before taking a jump to another level later, it was considered a jump followed by another jump. And a few said whole-heartedly "jump right in," yet in the next sentence revealed what they were doing or including that was "off plan." I guess we could refer to this group as "jumpers" with a little bit of tiptoe.

The important thing is to increase those actions and behaviors that are compatible with your goals so you get more consistent and just plain better at them. I promised a simple, proven plan for you to implement to realize your weight, health, energy, and body-shaping ideal. Now it's time to take what you like and make it your own. Where are you inspired to implement change?

When it comes to exercise, it's very effective to start with a goal you know you can achieve. What you strive for depends, in part, on your current level of fitness. Let's say you start with resistance training. Pick one, two, or three Fit Quickies, and practice them every other day for a week. The next week, add three new Fit Quickies. After a month, you'll have worked up to one of the endless varieties of full-body strengthening and shaping Fit Quickie routines I've provided and be ready to mix up some new combinations of your own. Set the timer so you get up from your work station and move your body every 45 minutes. Or work in 10 minutes of Fit Quickies at least once a day. You can alternate Fit Quickies with any other resistance-training program you enjoy. Then add another element of fitness to your healthy fitness plan piece by piece.

Whatever you choose to start with, commit to simply being more active every day, create a specific intention of being less sedentary, and support it with a plan of action. Quite quickly, you'll discover you have an active lifestyle, with all the benefits it brings. Never underestimate the physically restoring and mentally resurrecting power of moving your body.

One of the most successful strategies of changing your diet is to keep adding more of the foods you want to focus on to your daily diet. This crowds out less-nutritious, low-fiber, high-fat, and processed foods. Many people are highly successful by starting right there. Use the "Nutrition Principles" chapter as a guide to inspire you to fill your plate generously from the five food groups. At first you'll be astonished at how much food you get to eat and still get and stay trim. And believe me, you'll never tire of being able to be full without being fat. I never do.

If you're already at an intermediate or advanced level with your exercise and diet, perhaps you're ready to step up to a new challenge. And if you're already a champion with both yet need new to create more variety or balance in your workouts or food plan, now is the time.

It Takes All Three Pillars

Remember the three pillars from earlier in the book? Think of these three as the essential legs of your success tripod: fitness, food, and frame of mind. The truth is, when you get the food right, the fitness is so much easier. The dietary guide as I put together for you in the "Nutrition Principles" chapter combined with targeted body shapers and a little bit of cardio is what makes it so astonishingly simple for me to stay in shape—and shaped. Honoring the supreme importance of giving equal time to mastery of mind-set makes success in the physical—with food and fitness—so absolutely possible. With my food plan, the exercise prescription and tools for mind-set mastery, you have three winning tickets. Put them together, and you have a season pass.

Mastery doesn't mean "perfection." Mastery is a journey piloted by practice. And practicing specific behaviors, day after day, builds your tower of attainment. Mirror these same strategies of progressing success with each of the pillars.

Remember that without the guide of a vision, and your *why*, you're playing at a disadvantage. Find it and craft from it your goals and then plan and take specific actions that support them. Keep the principles of the "Motivation and Mind-Set for Success" chapter as your companions as you plan and navigate your path to mastery and success. All habit change demands motivation and ability. Set specific intentions for changes that you know are doable, such as a specific food to incorporate into your diet every day, or an activity of body or mind to practice regularly. This is how you make small additions that add up to big change. Cultivate the long stride only possible by take smaller specific steps.

Think of the changes you're making as an adventure—an adventure into better health, increased well-being, and a better body. Truly healthy living is a combination of conscious eating, regular exercise, and good attitude. Keep incorporating more healthy choices that support your goals, and allow them to edge out the less desirable. That way, you keep building on wins. Add the critical elements of patience, consistency, heart, and compassion for yourself. Your healthy choices will soon become your habits, and these habits will quickly become your healthy lifestyle. Before you know it, a healthy lifestyle will become your destiny.

APPENDIX
RESOURCES

The finish of this book doesn't mean the end of support from me—it's just the beginning. I've created and gathered multiple resources at my website, lanimuelrath.com. You'll find Fit Quickies video and audio downloads, Lani's Dessert Guided Relaxation, motivational programs, plant-based nutrition education and support, fitness assessment tools, archives of instructional and motivational articles, videos, recipes, training guides, and more here, all a few easy clicks from the home page. You'll discover options for special programs, coaching, and a newsletter for regular updates, with all the news for healthy fitness from me, the Plant-Based Fitness Expert.

To learn more, go to lanimuelrath.com. You can write to me at info@lanimuelrath.com.

Books and Journals

Here are some of my recommended favorite books as well as cited journals, if you'd like a little more information on anything I've presented in this book.

Antonello, Jean. *How to Become Naturally Thin by Eating More.* St. Paul, Minnesota: Heartland Book Co., 1989.

Barnard, Neal. *Reversing Diabetes.* New York: Rodale, 2007.

———. *Turn Off Your Fat Genes.* New York: Harmony, 2001.

Campbell, T. Colin, PhD, with Thomas M. Campbell II. *The China Study.* Dallas: BenBella Books, 2006.

Hever, Julieanna. *The Complete Idiot's Guide to Plant-Based Nutrition.* Indianapolis, Indiana: Alpha Books, 2011.

Lisle, Doug, and Alan Goldhamer. *The Pleasure Trap*. Summertown, Tennessee: Healthy Living Publications, 2003.

McDougall, John, and Mary McDougall. *The Starch Solution*. New York: Rodale Press, 2012.

McGonigal, Kelly, PhD. *The Willpower Instinct: How Self-Control Works, Why It Matters and What You Can Do to Get More of It*. New York: Avery, 2012.

Robbins, John. *Diet for a New America*. Toronto: Fitzhenry and Whiteside, 1987.

Exercise and Fit Quickies

Anders, Mark. "Glutes to the Max." *ACE FitnessMatters* (February 2006): 7–9.

———. "New Study Puts the Crunch on Ineffective Ab Exercises." *ACE FitnessMatters* (May/June 2001): 9–11.

Bauman, W. A., and Spungen, A. M. "Coronary Heart Disease in Individuals with Spinal Cord Injury: Assessment of Risk Factors." *Spinal Cord* 46, no. 7 (2008): 466–476.

Bemben, D. A., N. L. Fetters, M. G. Bemben, N. Nabavi, and E. T. Koh. "Musculoskeletal Responses to High- and Low-Intensity Resistance Training in Early Postmenopausal Women." *Medicine and Science in Sports and Exercise* 32, no. 11 (2000): 1,949–1,957.

Benke, Robert S. *Kinetic Anatomy, Second Edition*. Champaign, Illinois: Human Kinetics Inc., 2006.

Bey, Lional, and Marc T. Hamilton. "Suppression of Skeletal Muscle Lipoprotein Lipase Activity During Physical Inactivity: A Molecular Reason to Maintain Daily Low-Intensity Activity." *The Journal of Physiology* (September 2003): 551, 673–682.

Boehler, Brittany; J. Porcari, PhD; D. Kline, MS; C. Hendrix, PhD; and Carl Foster, PhD; with Mark Anders. "Best Triceps Exercises." *ACE Certified News* (August 2011): acefitness.org/certifiednewsarticle/1562/ace-sponsored-research-best-triceps-exercises.

Boreham C. A., R. A. Kennedy, M. H. Murphy, M. Tully, W. F. Wallace, and I. Young. "Training Effects of Short Bouts of Stair Climbing on Cardiorespiratory Fitness, Blood Lipids, and Homocysteine in Sedentary Young Women." *British Journal of Sports Medicine* 39, no. 9 (September 2005): 590–593.

Burd, N. A., C. Mitchell, T. Churchward-Venne, and Stuart M. Phillips. "Bigger Weights May Not Beget Bigger Muscles: Evidence from Acute Muscle Protein Synthetic Responses After Resistance Exercise." *Applied Physiology, Nutrition, and Metabolism* 37 (2012): 551–554.

Burd N. A., D. West, A. Staples, P. Atherton, J. Baker, et al. "Low-Load High Volume Resistance Exercise Stimulates Muscle Protein Synthesis More Than High-Load Low Volume Resistance Exercise in Young Men." *PLoS ONE* 5, no. 8 (2010): e12033.

Galati, Todd, MA. "ACE IFT Model for Cardiorespiratory Training: Phases 1–4." *ACE Certified News* (August 2010): acefitness.org/certifiednewsarticle/709/ace-ift-model-for-cardiorespiratory-training.

Garber, C. E., et al. "Quantity and Quality of Exercise for Developing and Maintaining Cardiorespiratory, Musculoskeletal, and Neuromotor Fitness in Apparently Healthy Adults: Guidance for Prescribing Exercise." *Medicine and Science in Sports and Exercise* 43, no. 7 (2011): 1,334–1,359.

Hamburg, N. M., C. J. McMackin, A. L. Huang, S. M. Shenouda, M. E. Widlansky, E. Schulz, et al. "Physical Inactivity Rapidly Induces Insulin Resistance and Microvascular Dysfunction in Healthy Volunteers." *Arteriosclerosis, Thrombosis, and Vascular Biology* 27, no. 12 (2007): 2,650–2,656.

Hamilton, Mark T., and Lionel Bay. "Suppression of Skeletal Muscle Lipoprotein Lipase Activity During Physical Inactivity: A Molecular Reason to Maintain Daily Low-Intensity Activity." *The Journal of Physiology* (September 1, 2003): 673–682.

Hamilton, Marc T., Deborah G. Hamilton, and Theodore W. Zderic. "Role of Low Energy Expenditure and Sitting in Obesity, Metabolic Syndrome, Type 2 Diabetes, and Cardiovascular Disease." *Diabetes* 56, no. 11 (November 2007): 2,655–2,667.

Harmon, N. M., and L. Kravitz. "The Effects of Music on Exercise." *IDEA Fitness Journal* 4, no. 8 (2007): 72–77.

Healy, Genevieve N., MPH; David W. Dunstan, PH; Jo Salmon, PHD; Ester Cerin, PHD; Jonathan E. Shaw, MD; Paul Z. Zimmet, MD; and Neville Owen, PHD. "Breaks in Sedentary Time: Beneficial Associations with Metabolic Risk." *Diabetes Care* 31, no. 4 (April 2008): 661–666.

Karageorghis, C. I., and P. C. Terry. "The Psychophysical Effects of Music in Sport and Exercise: A Review." *Journal of Sport Behavior* 20, no. 1 (1997): 54–68.

Karpinelli, Ralph N. "The Size Principal and a Critical Analysis of the Unsubstantiated Heavier-Is-Better Recommendation for Resistance Training." *Journal of Exercise Science and Fitness* 6, no. 2 (2008): 67–86.

Katch, F. I., P. M. Clarkson, W. Kroll, and T. McBride. "Effects of Sit-up Exercise Training on Adipose Cell Size and Adiposity." *Research Quarterly for Exercise and Sport* 55 (1984): 242–247.

Katzmarzyk, Peter T., Timothy S. Church, Cora L. Craig, and Claude Bouchard. "Sitting Time and Mortality from All Causes, Cardiovascular Disease, and Cancer." *Medicine and Science in Sports* 41, no. 5 (May 2009): 998–1,005.

Kravitz, Len, PhD, and Ken Fowler. "Perils of Poor Posture." *IDEA Fitness Journal* 8, no. 4 (April 2011): 18–21.

Murphy, M. H., and A. E. Hardman. "Training Effects of Short and Long Bouts of Brisk Walking in Sedentary Women." *Medicine and Science in Sports and Exercise* 30, no. 1 (January 1998): 152–157.

Murphy, M., A. Nevill, C. Neville, S. Biddle, and A. Hardman. "Accumulating Brisk Walking for Fitness, Cardiovascular Risk, and Psychological Health." *Medicine and Science in Sports and Exercise* 34, no. 9 (September 2002): 1,468–1,474.

Neumann, Donald A. *Kinesiology of the Muskuloskeletal System, Foundations for Rehabilitation.* St. Louis: Mosby Inc., 2002.

Owen, Neville, G. Healy, C. Matthews, and D. Dunstan. "Too Much Sitting: The Population-Health Science of Sedentary Behavior." *Science of Sedentary Behavior* 38, no. 3 (July 2010).

Persinger, R., C. Foster, M. Gibson, D. C. W. Fater, and J. P. Porcari. "Consistency of the Talk Test for Exercise Prescription." *Medicine and Science Sports and Exercise* 36, no. 9 (2004): 1,632–1,636.

Russell, B., D. Motlagh, and W. W. Ashley. "Form Follows Functions: How Muscle Shape Is Regulated by Work." *Journal of Applied Physiology* 88 (2000): 1,127–1,132.

Serwe, Katrina M., Ann M. Swartz, Teresa L. Hart, and Scott J. Strath. "Effectiveness of Long and Short Bout Walking on Increasing Physical Activity in Women." *Journal of Women's Health* 20, no. 2 (February 2011): 247–253.

Szmedra, L., and D. W. Bacharach. "Effect of Music on Perceived Exertion, Plasma Lactate, Norepinephrine and Cardiovascular Hemodynamics During Treadmill Running." *International Journal of Sports Medicine* 19, no. 1 (1998): 32–37.

Szabo, A., A. Small, and M. Leigh. "The Effects of Slow- and Fast-Rhythm Classical Music on Progressive Cycling to Voluntary Physical Exhaustion." *The Journal of Sports Medicine and Physical Fitness* 39, no. 3 (1999): 220–225.

Tremblay, M. S., R. C. Colley, T. J. Saunders, G. N. Healy, and N. Owen. "Physiological and Health Implications of a Sedentary Lifestyle." *Applied Physiology, Nutrition, and Metabolism* 35, no. 6 (December 2010): 725–740.

Yanagibori, R., K. Kondo, Y. Suzuki, K. Kawakubo, T. Iwamoto, H. Itakura, and A. Gunji. "Effect of 20 Days Bed Rest on the Reverse Cholesterol Transport System in Healthy Young Subjects." *Journal of Internal Medicine* 243 (1998): 307–312.

Zderic, Theodore W., and Marc T. Hamilton. "Physical Inactivity Amplifies the Sensitivity of Skeletal Muscle to the Lipid-Induced Downregulation of Lipoprotein Lipase Activity." *Journal of Applied Physiology* 100, no. 1 (January 2006): 249–257.

Diet and Nutrition

Bell, Elizabeth A., V. H. Castellanos, C. L. Pelkman, M. L. Thorwart, and B. J. Rolls. "Energy Density of Foods Affects Energy Intake in Normal-Weight Women." *American Journal of Clinical Nutrition* 67 (1998): 412–420.

Benelam, B. "Satiation, Satiety and Their Effects on Eating Behavior." *Nutrition Bulletin* 34, no. 2 (June 2009): 126–173.

Blundell, J. E., and V. J. Burley. "Satiation, Satiety and the Action of Fibre on Food Intake." *International Journal of Obesity* 11 (1987): 9–25.

Bray, G. A. "Afferent Signals Regulating Food Intake." *Proceedings of the Nutrition Society* 59, no. 3 (2000): 373–84.

Burley, V. J., A. W. Paul, and J. E. Blundell. "Influence of a High-Fibre Food (Myco-protein) on Appetite: Effects on Satiation (Within Meals) and Satiety (Following Meals)." *European Journal of Clinical Nutrition* 47, no. 6 (June 1993): 409–418.

Campbell, T. Colin. "Nutrition Fundamentals State of Health." T. Colin Campbell Foundation and TILS Articles, 2008.

Cotton, J. R., V. J. Burley, J. A. Weststrate, and J. E. Blundell. "Dietary Fat and Appetite: Similarities and Differences in the Satiating Effect of Meals Supplemented with Either Fat or Carbohydrate." *Journal of Human Nutrition and Diet* 20, no. 3 (June 2007): 186–199.

Deutsch, J. A. "The Role of the Stomach in Eating." *American Journal of Clinical Nutrition* 42, no. 5 Suppl. (1985): 1,040–1,043.

Duncan, K. H., J. A. Bacon, and R. L. Weinsier. "The Effects of High and Low Energy Density Diets on Satiety, Energy Intake, and Eating Time of Obese and Nonobese Subjects." *American Journal of Clinical Nutrition* 37 (1983): 763–767.

Drewnowski, A. "Energy Density, Palatability, and Satiety: Implications for Weight Control." *Nutrition Review* 56 (1998): 347–353.

Haber, G. B., K. W. Heaton, D. Murphy, and L. F. Burroughs. "Depletion and Disruption of Dietary Fibre. Effects on Satiety, Plasma-Glucose, and Serum-Insulin." *Lancet* 2, no. 8,040 (October 1, 1977): 679–682.

Heaton, K. W., S. N. Marcus, P. M. Emmett, and C. H. Bolton. "Particle Size of Wheat, Maize, and Oat Test Meals: Effects on Plasma Glucose and Insulin Responses and on the Rate of Starch Digestion in Vitro." *American Journal of Clinical Nutrition* 47, no. 4 (April 1988): 675–682.

Holt, S. H., H. J. Delargy, C. L. Lawton, and J. E. Blundell. "The Effects of High-Carbohydrate vs. High-Fat Breakfasts on Feelings of Fullness and Alertness, and Subsequent Food Intake." *International Journal of Food Science and Nutrition* 50, no. 1 (January 1999): 13–28.

Houpt, K. A. "Gastrointestinal Factors in Hunger and Satiety." *Neuroscience and Biobehavioral Reviews* 6, no. 2 (Summer 1982): 145–164.

Leary, M. R., et al. "Self-Compassion and Reactions to Unpleasant Self-Relevant Events: The Implications of Treating Oneself Kindly." *Journal of Personality and Social Psychology* 92, no. 5 (2007): 887–904.

Mickelsen, O., D. D. Makdani, R. H. Cotton, S. T. Titcomb, J. C. Colmey, and R. Gatty. "Effects of a High Fiber Bread Diet on Weight Loss in College-Age Males." *American Journal of Clinical Nutrition* 32, no. 8 (August 1979): 1,703–1,709.

Paintal, A. S. "A Study of Gastric Stretch Receptors. Their Role in the Peripheral Mechanism of Satiation of Hunger and Thirst." *Journal of Physiology* 126, no. 2 (November 29, 1954): 255–270.

Read, N. "Role of Gastrointestinal Factors in Hunger and Satiety in Man." *Proceedings of the Nutrition Society* 51 (1992): 7–11.

Read, N., S. French, and K. Cunningham. "The Role of the Gut in Regulating Food Intake in Man." *Nutrition Reviews* 52, no. 1 (1994): 1–10.

Rolls, B. J., E. A. Bell, V. H. Castellanos, M. Chow, C. L. Pelkman, and M. L. Thorwart. "Energy Density but Not Fat Content of Foods Affected Energy Intake in Lean and Obese Women." *American Journal of Clinical Nutrition* 69 (1999): 863–871.

Rolls, B. J., S. Kim-Harris, M. W. Fischman, R. W. Foltin, T. H. Moran, and S. A. Stoner. "Satiety After Preloads with Different Amounts of Fat and Carbohydrate: Implications for Obesity." *American Journal of Clinical Nutrition.* 60 (1994): 476–487.

Seagle, H. M., B. M. Davy, G. Grunwald, and J. O. Hill. "Energy Density of Self Reported Food Intake: Variation and Relationship to Other Food Components." *Obesity Research* 5 (Suppl., 1997): S87.

Stubbs, R. J., C. G. Harbron , P. R. Murgatroyd, and A. M. Prentice. "Covert Manipulation of Dietary Fat and Energy Density: Effect on Substrate Flux and Food Intake in Men Eating Ad Libitum." *American Journal of Clinical Nutrition* 62 (1995): 316–329.

Stubbs, R. J., P. Ritz, W. A. Coward, and A. M. Prentice. "Covert Manipulation of the Ratio of Dietary Fat to Carbohydrate and Energy Density: Effect on Food Intake and Energy Balance in Free-Living Men Eating Ad Libitum." *American Journal of Clinical Nutrition* 62 (1995): 330–337.

Whybrow, S. "Energy Density and Weight Control. Food, Diet and Obesity." *Woodhead Publishing in Food Science and Technology*. Cambridge, UK: Woodhead Publishing Limited, 2005.

Motivation, Mind-Set, and Willpower

Adams, C. E., and M. R. Leary. "Promoting Self-Compassionate Attitudes Toward Eating Among Restrictive and Guilty Eaters." *Journal of Social and Clinical Psychology* 26, no. 10 (2007): 1,120–1,144.

Appelhans, B. M., and L. J. Luecken. "Heart Rate Variability As an Index of Regulated Emotional Responding." *Review of General Psychology* 10, no. 3 (2006): 229–240.

Barton, J., and J. Pretty. "What Is the Best Dose of Nature and Green Exercise for Improving Mental Health? A Multi-study Analysis." *Environmental Science and Technology* 44, no. 10 (2010): 3,947–3,955.

Bowen, S., and A. Marlatt. "Surfing the Urge: Brief Mindfulness-Based Intervention for College Student Smokers." *Psychology of Addictive Behavior* 23, no. 4 (2009): 666–671.

Baumeister, Roy, and K. D. Vohs. "Self-Regulation, Ego Depletion, and Motivation." *Social and Personality Psychology Compass* 1, no 1. (November 2007): 115–128.

Frederickson, Fabienne. Inner Game of Abundance Mindset Retreat, 2011. client attraction. com.

Figner, Berndl, D. Knoch, E. J. Johnson, A. R. Kroschl, S. Lisanby, E. Fehr, and E. Weber. "Lateral Prefrontal Cortex and Self-Control in Intertemporal Choice." *Nature Neuroscience* 13 (2010):538–539.

Gailliot, M. T., et al. "Self-Control Relies on Glucose As a Limited Energy Source: Willpower Is More Than a Metaphor." *Journal of Personality and Social Psychology* 92, no. 2 (2007): 325–336.

Hansen, C. J., L. C. Stevens, and J. R. Coast. "Exercise Duration and Mood State: How Much Is Enough to Feel Better?" *Health Psychology* 20, no. 4:, 267–275.

Heatherton, T. F., J. Polivy, and C. P. Herman. "Dietary Restraint: Some Current Findings and Speculations." *Psychology of Addictive Behavior* 4, no. 2 (1990): 100–106.

Hölzel, B. K., J. Carmody, M. Vangel, C. Congleton, S. M. Yerramsetti, T. Gard, and S. W. Lazar. "Mindfulness Practice Leads to Increases in Regional Brain Gray Matter Density." *Psychiatry Research* 191, no. 1 (January 30, 2011): 36–43.

Leonard, George. *Mastery: The Keys to Success and Long-Term Fulfillment.* New York: Penguin Group, 1991.

Oaten, M., and K. Cheng. "Longitudinal Gains in Self-Regulation Through Regular Exercise." *British Journal of Health Psychology* 11 (2006): 717–733.

Sapolsky, R. M. "The Frontal Cortex and the Criminal Justice System." *Philosophical Transactions of the Royal Society of London, Series B, Biological Science* 359 (2004): 1,787–1,796.

Song, H. S., and P. M. Lehrer. "The Effects of Specific Respiratory Rates on Heart Rate and Heart Rate Variability." *Applied Psychophysiology and Biofeedback* 28 (2003): 13–23.

DVD

Lisle, Doug. *The Continuum of Evil: How to Lose Weight Without Losing Your Mind.* drmcdougall.com/store_continuum_of_evil.html.

INDEX

Q-R

T

U